To Lloyd Duplantis,
without whose inspiration this book would not be in
your hands.

Full Disclosure:

Major revisions to this book were made using pens supplied by the pharmaceutical industry.

Finally, someone had figured out how to poison a person. You caught by the title of the book, I hope, that I'm a pharmacist, and anyone in my or any of the related medical professions should totally know how to poison a person if they want to. It's not nearly as hard as you might think. Yet more than once over the years I've read a story about a nurse, a doctor, a veterinarian or even a dentist who would try to off someone in a totally inappropriate way. They should all know morphine or any other narcotic, while effective for putting a person to permanent sleep, produces a distinct set of symptoms in your target and is detectable post-mortem. Same with arsenic and most of your other traditional chemical killers. I would read news accounts of people in the professions who tried to poison people using these agents and I would heckle them, much the same way you might heckle an outfielder who muffed a routine fly ball. "You suck doctor!!!! Did you really not think anyone would notice how your ex-wife's muscles all seized up and not think you might have slipped her some strychnine? BOOOOOOOOOOOOO!!!!!!"

That's why a friend of mine insisted I watch an episode of *Desperate Housewives* a few years back I guess. I don't watch a lot of TV, but he seemed to think I would get something out of this show. He was not mistaken. When I saw the potassium I'm pretty sure I let out an audible cheer. Finally, someone had figured out how to poison a person. And it was a pharmacist, albeit a fictional one. I felt a little pride in my profession, as once again we were showing the rest of the medical field who was the drug expert. In your face morphine nurse!!

So yeah, I'm a little different from your stereotypical pharmacist I guess.

For most of my career if you had asked me why I chose this profession I wouldn't have been able to tell you. I may have entered my career a bit twisted, but twenty years behind the pharmacy counter has turned my mind into the most Gordian of knots. Not twisted in an evil way mind you, like that *Desperate Housewives* pharmacist who killed a customer in order to improve his chances of being able to score with the widow, or the real world pharmacist in Kansas City who once diluted chemotherapy meds in order to improve his bottom line. No, I'm more of a send you to the wrong aisle when you ask me where the paper plates are kinda guy. Harmless really, but very capable of messing with you. I'll always make sure you get the right medicine and that all your questions get answered, but more than likely I secretly hate you. I'm an anti-socialite in a people oriented profession. Not a recipe for mental stability really. I wonder a lot how I got into this place.

I blame a little plastic motorcycle and Nuprin.

I can honestly say that Nuprin changed my life. I was in the pimply faced, awkward phase that is junior high, a lump of clay ready to be molded and shaped and nerdy enough that I found it fascinating that one of the magical preparations that had always been kept away from me, three feet higher and a good five yards back from anywhere I could be, was now in my very hands.

It was little.

It was yellow.

It was different.

It was ibuprofen, and in 1984, Nuprin, along with its partner Advil, took the pain relieving world by storm. I became drunk on the taste of drug knowledge that learning about Nuprin had given me, and was still fascinated with the discovery that ibuprofen not only relieved pain but also was an anti-inflammatory when I saw a classified ad that listed a pharmacist's salary.

"They make how much?" I thought.

"I could do that."

My fate was sealed. Three years later I applied to pharmacy school. Many kids since then have asked me for tips or tricks or other types of guidance on how to become a pharmacist. We do make decent money, and it's not as hard as you might think. Here's the deal:

The process will start sometime around your junior year of high school:

1) If you see a class with chemistry and/or biology in the name, take it.

Try to learn something.

2) If you are in a band, any band making any kind of music, drop out, as you will have to eliminate all right brain creative and artistic function. This does not apply to marching bands however, as i) marching bands don't make music, and ii) mindlessly following orders will help you immensely in your career choice.

3) Start thinking about colleges. Forget the Ivy League, the big state school known only for its football team will do you just fine.

High School Senior year:

1) Take them chemistry and biology classes like you are crazy for the science.

2) Drop your creative writing class.

3) Start asking people if they have their prescription insurance card with them. Practice being incredibly annoyed when they don't.

4) Visit some college campuses and look for one with a lot of middle class snot-ass kids who never got the memo they're not rich. Lots of Asians are also a good sign.

5) If you do not graduate in the top 10% of your high school class, immediately kill yourself, as your life is over. Or join the military.

Pre-pharmacy college years:

1) Foolishly show up on campus under the impression you are going to learn something about drugs sometime soon. Wash away your disappointment in a river of beer.

2) Master the process of counting by fives while waving a short metal stick from right to left.

3) More chemistry! Remember, you are a chemistry loving fool!

4) Start negotiations with Satan over the price of your soul. He will not offer enough to cover tuition.

5) Imagine for a few hours what it would be like to want to help people. This will help you write the required essay when the time comes to apply for pharmacy school.

6) Develop an intense hatred for the business major that lives across the hall from you. The same one that knocks on your door EVERY FUCKING NIGHT TO ASK IF YOU WANT TO GO BAR HOPPING! JESUS H. CHRIST DON'T THESE FUCKING BUSINESS MAJORS EVER HAVE TO LOOK AT THE INSIDE OF A BOOK AT ANY TIME IN THEIR COLLEGE CAREER? The experience you have with business majors during college will set the stage

7

for relations with your district manager or hospital administrator throughout your working life.

Pharmacy School:

1) Congratulations! The second an actual college of pharmacy accepts your application, you never have to worry about grades again. Simply remember this GPA formula; 2.0 = $110k/year

2) Show up for your first day of work as a pharmacy intern, feel the door close behind you, and as the chill settles into your spine, know that all joy is gone from your existence, forever.

3) Take a philosophy class. You need this class in order to graduate. No one working for the University seems to know why.

4) Still more chemistry. And they still haven't taught you how to make crystal meth.

5) Realize that gin mixed in orange juice really doesn't taste all that bad when you have no money. Lose your virginity to that girl in pharmaceutics lab who wears the coke bottle glasses and never talks.

6) You will have no recollection of anything that happens between mid-April of your last year of school and the end of your college career. Memory will fade back in as you walk across a stage wearing a gown and suffering from the worst hangover of your life. The president of the University will hand you a document you assume is your diploma. Upon opening it 5 days later, you see it is actually a student loan repayment schedule. Your first payment is already a week late.

7) Attempt to cram everything you've learned over the last six years into the three months you have to ready yourself for the pharmacy licensure exam. Realize you've learned nothing, rekindle the relationship with coke-bottle chick so you can sit next to her during the test and copy her answers.

8) Find out that yes, the condom did break and coke bottle chick is absolutely thrilled to be starting a family. Marriage certificate is issued on the same day pharmacy license arrives in the mail, officially documenting the end of your life

You may find this overly cynical. After all, you went into this to help people, and for the money. Now you're a respected professional, in one of the most respected occupations in the country. You've been told you're going to be an integral part of the clinical decision making health care team, and you're raring to go. Great. Here's what to expect when you settle into your job at the drugstore. This was a typical day at my typical pharmacy. All I did was keep a little notebook by my work computer so I wouldn't forget the details:

The day started with the following actual question from an actual customer who required a doctor's authorization for a prescription refill on his Vicodin, a narcotic painkiller. He was wearing a Superman t-shirt.

"My doctor's not there today, do you think they'll call it in by this afternoon?"

I didn't try to explain why, I just told the nice customer probably not. I've learned trying to explain why only makes it worse.

I did manage to get a hold of a doctor who was in the office to let him know he prescribed penicillin to a patient whose "tongue swole up real bad" the last time he took penicillin. The nice doctor switched the prescription and the customer thanked me for my efforts by complaining how much more expensive the new med was. I tried to explain that anaphylactic shock is remembered long after price is forgotten, but the nice customer was in a bargain hunting mood. The new med was erythromycin. It cost $3 more.

Superman called back in a couple hours, asked for me by name, and waited five minutes on hold until I could get the phone so he could ask:

"Has my doctor called yet?"

Me: "No."

Customer: "OK, I think I'll drive over there."

Mid afternoon brought the following conversation:

Customer: "This new medicine is 100 milligrams. Can I switch back to my old one?"

Me: "Well, how has your blood pressure been on this new medicine?"

Customer: "It's been good. That other med never really got it under control."

Me: "Is that why your doctor switched you?"

Customer: "No, the other one made my tongue swell up."

The tongue swelling thing seems to come in cycles.

Me: "So......your old medicine never really got your blood pressure under control, and made your tongue swell. Why do you want to switch back?"

Customer: "This new medicine is 100 milligrams. My old medicine was 20 milligrams"

This was a serious issue to this person. I tried to explain and wished for the simplicity of a conversation with Superman.

Be careful what you wish for. He called back to let me know he was in the parking lot of his doctor's office but couldn't find the entrance.

This was followed by a call from a customer who told us they accidentally took the store's bathroom key home with them. This key is attached to a piece of wood probably half a yard long and colored bright blue. You can see it from a mile away and fit it into probably less than 5% of purses ever made. Not to mention a bathroom key is the type of thing you really don't want to handle any more than necessary. Yet someone took it home. I thought to myself that we had reached the rock bottom of stupidity.

I should have remembered you can never go broke betting on stupid. Five minutes later I saw the bathroom key in the break room, right where it belonged. The only thing dumber than taking home a store's bathroom key is thinking you took it home when you didn't.

Superman never got his Vicodin, and that's what will await you day after day, week after week, year after year on the other side of pharmacy school. Remember that while you're in college getting pumped full of the data you'll need to make critically important clinical decisions. Remember Superman.

I don't totally blame Nuprin though. While it steered me towards a particular profession, looking back I'm pretty sure it was the little plastic stunt motorcycle that set the tone for my life.

I don't even know why I asked for the little plastic stunt motorcycle that first year. It was named after a famous daredevil of the era of my boyhood, but I'm pretty sure I never actually saw the guy do any of his televised jumps. It was probably the fourth or fifth thing on my Christmas list, but the only one I didn't get. I thought that was a little weird, and made sure to put the little plastic stunt motorcycle at the top of my greed list the next year. Again, every single thing on my list, and then some, appeared under the tree come Christmas, but no little plastic stunt motorcycle. I thought maybe Santa was fucking with me.

The third year the little plastic stunt motorcycle was my top priority. I started lobbying weeks in advance. One time after a huge snowstorm I shoveled the driveway without being asked. Dad yelled at me because I did it in my tennis shoes. Dad always had a thing about proper winter footwear. For the last time in my life, I made an effort to be good and kind and caring. The third year was gonna be make or break for the little plastic stunt motorcycle, and I pulled out all the stops.

You know what happened. I got a Bionic Man rocket ship that turned into an operating table. Whose idea was it to even design such a thing? I mean, would you want the space shuttle to turn into a giant surgical suite for some reason? My spirit was broken, but I continued to ask for the little plastic stunt motorcycle, its place lower and lower on my Christmas list each year until it was replaced with a request for The Beatles White Album. I didn't get that either.

A couple years ago I finally asked my Mom why I never got the little plastic stunt motorcycle. "Oh, I don't remember" was the reply. The mystery of the little plastic motorcycle would never be solved. A part of me would never be at peace.

I explained this to one of my technicians at work once when she asked me why I was so warped and she got a good chuckle out of the story, but the cashier had not a clue what I was talking about. As I tried to explain the concept of the little plastic stunt motorcycle set to the cashier, all those old feelings came back to me. It was like I was lobbying my Mom all over again, telling her how incredibly cool this toy was, and how cool I would be if only I could have it.

Then I realized. I'm an adult now, with my own money and control over my own purchasing decisions. Betcha I could totally find a little plastic stunt motorcycle on eBay. I decided as soon as the long work weekend was over, I was gonna set aside some time to find me a little plastic stunt motorcycle.

Of course that's when the bastard the motorcycle was named after decided to die, promptly sending the price of a little plastic stunt motorcycle through the roof. I poured myself a giant dry martini, entered that magical buzz state where only gin can take you, pondered the situation, and after 30 years, it hit me.

That tone of voice. That my mom had when she said she couldn't remember. It was the exact same tone she uses when she doesn't want to talk about something. Dad had some sort of problem with that daredevil. I can't believe it took me this long to realize. I bet Dad thought the daredevil was gay. Jesus it all makes sense now. However, when you're on the young side of 10 years old, a little plastic stunt motorcycleless Christmas repeated 3 years in a row can set up a person for a lifetime of going through the motions and never expecting a payoff. The perfect mindset, actually, for a worklife full of people in Superman costumes asking for Vicodin refills. I understood, and accepted the curse of the daredevil.

You may have changed your impression of me from "cynical" to "cynic" by this point, but I prefer the term realist. I also think you'll appreciate my realism as I tell you the most important thing I've learned behind the pharmacy counter. Turn the page.

Why Your Prescription Takes So Damn Long To Fill:

It's the most common question I get from my perch behind the pharmacy counter, and the one most likely to make my head explode. I have a sinking feeling that if most people think about their pharmacist at all, it's because they're wondering why their prescription is taking so damn long to fill, and if you're standing at the bookstore leafing through this right now, there's a good chance once you find out the answer, you'll just put this book back and never buy it. I'm gonna take a chance though, because I retain a spark of hope for humanity. Here's why... your prescription takes so damn long to fill:

You come to the counter. I am on the phone with a drunk dude who wants the phone number to the grocery store next door. After I instruct him on the virtues of 411, you tell me your doctor was to phone in your prescription to me. Your doctor hasn't, and you're unwilling to wait until he does. Being in a generous mood, I call your doctors office and am put on hold for 5 minutes, then informed that your prescription was phoned in to my competitor on the other side of town. Phoning the competitor, I am immediately put on hold for 5 minutes before speaking to a clerk, who puts me back on hold to wait for the pharmacist. Your prescription is then transferred to me, and now I have to get the two phone calls that have been put on hold while this was being done. Now I return to the counter to ask if we've ever filled prescriptions for you before. For some reason, you think that "for you" means "for your cousin" and you answer my question with a "yes", whereupon I go the computer and see you are not on file.

The phone rings.

You have left to do something very important, such as browse through the monster truck magazines, and do not hear the three PA announcements requesting that you return to the pharmacy. You return eventually, expecting to pick up the finished prescription.....

The phone rings.

......only to find out that I need to ask your address, phone number, date of birth, if you have any allergies and insurance coverage. You tell me you're allergic to codeine. Since the prescription is for Vicodin, a narcotic painkiller which is a relative of codeine, I ask you what exactly codeine did to you when you took it. You say it made your stomach hurt. Every medicine on the market will make someone's stomach hurt, and if it made your stomach hurt before, it may or may not make your stomach hurt again. I roll my eyes and write down "no known allergies" You tell me......

The phone rings.

.....you have insurance and spend the next 5 minutes looking for your card. You give up and expect me to be able to file your claim anyway. I call my competitor and am immediately put on hold. Upon reaching a human, I ask them what insurance they have on file for you. I get the information and file your claim, which is rejected because you changed jobs 6 months ago. An asshole barges his way to the counter to ask where the bread is.

The phone rings.

I inform you that the insurance the other pharmacy has on file for you isn't working. You produce a card in less than 10 seconds that you seemed to be unable to find before. What you were really doing was hoping your old insurance would still work because it had a lower copay. Your new card prominently displays the logo of Blue Cross of Mystery, and even though Blue Cross of Mystery does in fact handle millions of prescription claims every year, for the group you belong to, the claim should go to a company called Innovative Fictional Pharmacy Solutions, whose logo is nowhere on the card.

The phone rings.

A lady comes to the counter wanting to know why the cherry flavored antacid works better than the lemon cream flavored antacid. What probably happened is that she had a milder case of heartburn when she took the cherry flavored brand, as they both use the exact same ingredient in the same strength. She will not be satisfied though until I confirm her belief that the cherry flavored brand is the superior product. I file your claim with Innovative Fictional Pharmacy Solutions, who rejects it because you had a 30 day supply of Vicodin filled 15 days ago at another pharmacy. You swear to me on your mother's....

The phone rings.

.......life that you did not have a Vicodin prescription filled recently. I call Innovative Fictional Pharmacy Solutions and am immediately placed on hold. The most beautiful woman on the planet walks by and notices not a thing. She has never talked to a pharmacist and never will. Upon reaching a human at Innovative Fictional Pharmacy Solutions, I am informed that the Vicodin prescription was indeed filled at another of my competitors. When I tell you this, you say you got hydrocodone there, not Vicodin. Hydrocodone is the generic name for Vicodin. Another little part of me dies.

The phone rings.

It turns out that a few days after your doctor wrote your last prescription, he told you to take it more frequently, meaning that what Innovative Fictional Pharmacy Solutions thought was a 30-day supply is indeed a 15 day supply with the new instructions. I call your doctor's office to confirm this and am immediately placed on hold. I call Innovative Fictional Pharmacy Solutions to get an override and am immediately placed on hold. My laser printer has a paper jam. It's time for my tech to go to lunch. Innovative Fictional Pharmacy Solutions issues the override and your claim goes though. Your insurance saves you 85 cents off the regular price of the prescription.

The phone rings.

At the cash register you sign....

The phone rings.

......the acknowledgement that you received a copy of my HIPAA policy and that I offered the required OBRA counseling for new prescriptions. HIPAA is an acronym for a federal law called "The Health Insurance Portability and Accountability Act of 1996 " It makes it illegal for me to share your health information with anyone except under certain defined circumstances. OBRA is shorthand for "The Omnibus Budget Reconciliation Act of 1990" It mandates that I offer to go over the uses, side effects, and other information with you when you pick up your new prescription. Only in Washington, D.C. does "insurance portability" mean "defining when you can share information" and "budget reconciliation" mean "talk to customers about their prescription." You remark that you're glad that your last pharmacist told you shouldn't take over the counter Tylenol along with the Vicodin, and that the acetaminophen you're taking instead seems to be working pretty well. I break the news to you that Tylenol is simply a brand name for acetaminophen and you don't believe me. Another part of me dies. You fumble around for two minutes looking for your checkbook and spend another two minutes making out a check for eight dollars and sixty seven cents. You ask why the tablets look different than those you got at the other pharmacy. I explain that they are from a different manufacturer. Tomorrow you'll be back to tell me they don't work as well.

Now imagine this wasn't you at all, but the person who dropped off their prescription three people ahead of you, and you'll start to have an idea why.....your prescription takes so damn long to fill.

Now that I cleared that up I have a better question for you. Why does it take you so damn long to pick up a prescription? Seriously. All you have to do is give me your goddamn money and walk away. Those are the only requirements you have to meet. Which means you have a hell of a lot of chutzpah asking what took me so long. There's no law that says you must take 5 minutes to make out a check. As a matter of fact, it's perfectly legal for you to make out most of your check ahead of time, before you even approach the counter. If I tried to start evaluating potential drug interactions before you even presented me with a prescription, you might have a case for putting me in jail. So back the hell off.

You are also under no obligation to answer your phone the second it goes off while you are at the counter. I, however, am expected to take calls not only from your sorry ilk through the beginning, middle, and end of the prescription filling process, but from unimportant schleps like nurses and

14

doctors with questions of the type that can't be answered by reading your prescription label.

Which seem to be the only type of questions you can come up with. I love the "grab the bottle while simultaneously asking a question that can only be answered by looking at the bottle" maneuver. That speeds things up. Making both of us wait for you to put the goddamn bottle back down so I can tell you how many refills you have left after you realize you can't read the label that's been in front of your face for 30 seconds makes things nice and quick. Your commitment to speed in your own life only serves to motivate me to ask myself what I can do to make the prescription filling process faster.

Nothing. That's what I can do you ass. You however, could speed things along quite nicely by not treating me telling you your copay amount as the beginning of a negotiating session. I am not a car dealer. When I tell you how much your insurance company has determined your share of the cost of your prescription will be, you have two choices. 1) Accept it and pony up or 2) Don't pay it and go away. If you choose #2, I can return your prescription to you, but haggling will only rob us both of time we can never get back, and will never, ever, result in you paying one penny less. I don't care if it was $5 last time, I don't care what the status is of your deductible, and if I did, which let me say again that I don't, I would be powerless to change how much you owe me right now.

It also helps when you decide you have insurance only after you hear how expensive your prescription will be. Nice and quick that'll make things.

Have you finished making out that check yet? Didn't think so.

They called me The Drugnazi at the first place I made a living filling prescriptions. You now have an idea why. Jesus I wish my parents just would have gotten me that motorcycle.

The Answer To The Second Most Common Question I Get Behind The Counter. Your Prescription Costs So Much Because Drug Companies Are Out To Screw You.

I lied when I said the only time you think of me is when you're wondering why your prescription takes so long to fill. I also enter your mind when you want to know why your prescription costs so much. Fine. You want to know why your prescriptions cost so much? I'll tell you. Because for 20 years after they find a potentially marketable product, drug companies can charge you whatever they want, because that product will be covered by a patent. And you'll pay it. It's really not any more complicated than that.

Now how many of you just said something about how incredibly expensive it is for pharmaceutical manufacturers to do research and development, how they have to cover the costs of all the products that don't pan out, yadda yadda yadda.......?? I know some of you did. Every year since we decided it would be a hoot to put an actor in charge of running the country we have become a little more willing to toe the corporate line. Let me tell you a story though. A story about eardrops. A story that is 100% true.

Some of you may be familiar with Auralgan. It's a pain relieving prescription ear drop that's been around since the time of Moses. After Wyeth, the company that brought Auralgan to market sometime before the last ice age, lost its patent on the product, other manufacturers started making generic equivalents. As competition developed, the price of the generic Auralgans fell through the floor. This is the way these things usually go. The price of the generic Auralgans eventually fell so much that Wyeth stopped making the name brand. No one noticed. By that point Wyeth had lost so much market share it wasn't worth their while anymore. Doctors, however, were still used to writing the word "Auralgan" on their prescriptions. It is much easier to write than "antipyrine and benzocaine"

Enter Deston Therapeutics.

Deston Therapeutics had an ingenious plan to hit the big time. They would buy the rights to the name "Auralgan" from Wyeth, change the formula, and then start selling the new formula under the old name. Remember all those doctors who were still in the habit of writing "Auralgan" on a prescription pad? Well even though most of them had no idea about any changes, once that new formula hit the market, if I filled an Auralgan prescription the way I've filled it for years, I filled it wrong. There was no generic for the new Auralgan.

The price? $214.99. That wasn't a typo. The name that led to a cheap as dirt prescription 5 years ago will now set you back more than two Benjamin's.

Of course you do get the addition of acetic acid, which acts an anti-bacterial agent. It's also known as vinegar. I'm not making this up. Deston Therapeutics added some vinegar to an established product and raised the price by a factor of 14.

That must have taken a lot of research.

Let me end this story by saying don't ever put vinegar in your ear unless your doctor tells you to.

The story of Auralgan is an extreme one, but only mildly surprising to me by the time it happened in April of 2008. Because by April of 2008, I had had almost 20 years of inoculation to the tactics Big Pharma uses to separate you and your money, and the "just different enough to get a new patent" tactic has long been a mainstay of Big Pharma's money raising plans.

Here's a bit of organic chemistry you can use to make a mint in the drug business. Most biologically active compounds come in different forms, or "isomers." Put your hands up in front of your face. See how they are the same, but when you slide one in front of the other, they look different? Isomers are like that. Usually only one isomer is responsible for a drug's effects. Think of a lock and key and how you need a particular shape to open a lock, then look at your hands again.

How will this make you billions? Easy. If you hold the patent for a drug, somewhere around the 17th or 18th year of patent protection, all you need to do is come out with a product that is the biologically active isomer of your med, as opposed to the mixture of each isomer you originally marketed. You then call it something different, pretend like it's a brand new drug, and get a brand new patent. The anti-ulcer medicine Nexium, for example, ($173 for a 30 day supply of the most common strength according to drugstore.com) is simply one isomer of Prilosec ($22 for an over the counter generic). Dexilant ($130) is the active isomer of Prevacid ($20 and over the counter) Same deal with the anti-allergy meds Xyzal ($99) and Zyrtec ($10). And while there was research involved in unearthing this whole isomer business, I will point out it was done long ago. Generations ago actually, and it has long since been paid for. So why do Nexium, Dexilant, and Xyzal cost so much? Because as long as someone holds a patent for them, they can charge as much as they want.

And you'll pay it.

The oldest trick in the book however, may be the "XR" trick. Also known as the "CR, XL, or CD" sleight of hand. Here's how it works:

Again, somewhere around year, oh, 17 or 18 of patent protection, the research department of a drug manufacturer produces a breakthrough that allows a medicine to be dosed less frequently, let's say once a day as opposed to two or three times a day. It is amazing how these types of breakthroughs usually come in the years right before a patent expires. The drug manufacturer then gets a new patent covering the new delivery technology, and markets the old medicine in a new "eXtended Release, Continuous Release, or Continuous Delivery" form. I never heard what the "XL" is supposed to stand for. Perhaps it's the Roman numeral for the factor of increased profit the drug manufacturer expects if they can convince doctors to write for that version of the med instead of the newly available generic.

Of course you can make an argument that having to take your medicine less frequently is of some value, and you wouldn't be wrong. I'll let you decide for yourself though, the value of Paxil CR, a version of the common anti-depressant paroxetine. Generic paroxitine is dosed once a day and usually costs less than $10 a month. Paxil CR, on the other hand, will probably run you more than $120 for a 30 day supply, and is dosed....once a day. I'm not making that up. I never had a sales rep show up to explain to me the advantage of Paxil CR, perhaps because they were too embarrassed to show their face.

Pharmaceutical sales reps, by the way, are quite often stunningly gorgeous   women. My dentist, whose daughter was a college cheerleader, once told me more than one drug company sent their corporate recruiters after the cheerleading squad. She also told me that she found the prospect of a doctor learning all he knew about a medicine from her daughter to be frightening.

Those of you who worship at the altar of the free market are probably blue in the face by this point, or at least those of you who worship at the altar of the free market and don't have to pay full price for your prescriptions. "Dammit Drugnazi!" you're probably saying, "It costs a lot of money to develop a new medicine! Money doesn't grow on trees and these companies have to get their money back!!"

You're right. It does cost a lot of money to develop a new drug. About half as much as it does to market it. That's according to work published in 2008 by two researchers at York University in Toronto named Marc-André Gagnon and Joel Lexchin. All those commercials showing perfect, happy, people taking Wonderpill™ and implying that you too could be perfect and happy if only you would ask your doctor if Wonderpill™ is right for you? All the print advertisements you see? The Viagra race car? They're not free. They cost money. And money doesn't grow on trees you know. Remember that the next time you're giving me half of your next week's paycheck.

Also think about how no other country in the world pays as much for prescription medicines as we do. People in the United Kingdom, Germany, Japan, The Netherlands, Canada, Iceland, Greenland, Finland, pretty much any other land, they all pay a fraction of what you did the last time you saw me. Sucker.

Those free market worshipers I mentioned earlier are probably purple by now. More than likely ranting at high volume about how the United States has the best health care in the world, and how American quality health care doesn't come cheap.

Do we have the best health care in the world? Again, I'll let you decide:

-The United States has fewer doctors, fewer nurses, and fewer hospital beds per capita than the average country in the Organization for Economic Co-Operation and Development. Maybe by "best health care in the world" the ranters mean "fewer people providing health care"

-Rates of chronic disease are significantly higher among middle-aged people in the United States (before they are eligible for Medicare) than in that den of socialized medicine, the United Kingdom. The rate of diabetes is twice as high. Heart disease, 57% higher. Lung disease, 29% higher. Cancer.......73% higher. Maybe by "best health care in the world" the ranters mean "more people that need health care"

-37 countries have a higher life expectancy than the United States. Including Cuba, Chile, The United Arab Emirates, Costa Rica, Cyprus, and Malta. Maybe by "best health care in the world" the ranters mean "more people who die sooner"

If you're still on the fence I'll tell you that the World Health Organization set about ranking the world's healthcare systems in 2000, and put the United States 37th. Right behind Costa Rica. Granted, a lot has probably changed since 2000. Your insurance co-pays have probably gone up. If you still have insurance that is. And you'll probably wait longer for a doctor's appointment or in the Emergency Room than you would have back then.

The right-wing ranters are right about one thing though. American quality health care doesn't come cheap. There is one area of health care where the American system clearly leads the world. Spending! Here's a nice little factoid for those of you who like to think of yourselves as guardians of our taxpayer dollars. In the US, about 45% of the total amount spent on health care is paid for with government dollars. Our Canadian friends use government funds to foot the bill for about 70% of all health care in that country. And use fewer government dollars per person to do it.

Are you getting this? Canada runs an entire health care system, for everyone, for less per person than we spend on just Medicare and Medicaid. So does France. And Japan. You'll find Japan at the top of the list of life expectancy by country. The UK that so kicks our ass in chronic disease prevention does it while spending about 60% less per person than we do.

Tell me again why I'm supposed to be afraid of socialized medicine?

Now that I've either shut up the right wing ranters among you or they have died of self-asphyxiation, I'll drop the big bombshell. Drug companies have done more than play the "XR" trick. They've done more than run commercials during "60 Minutes" trying to convince you you have restless legs syndrome or Social Anxiety Disorder. There have been times when drug companies have manipulated, some might even say falsified, the very science most of us believe is the foundation of their existence.

How I Lost The Blind Faith In Science Five Years Of Pharmacy School Had Given Me.

Who here likes breast cancer? No one I bet. Who here would stand in the way of a therapy that would decrease the breast cancer rate almost instantaneously by almost 10%? No one I bet. Wow! Can you imagine? 20,000 cases of breast cancer a year gone with the wave of a magic wand. How much do you think a therapy like that would be worth? How much would you pay to reduce your risk of breast cancer by 10%?

What if I told you you didn't have pay anything? That breast cancer rates went down by almost 10% from 2000 to 2004 and it didn't cost one thin dime. Some people might be thinking Big Pharma discovered a breakthrough breast cancer medicine and was so excited about the potential to reduce human suffering that they gave it away for free, much the way Dr. Jonas Salk thought it would be unconscionable to profit from the polio vaccine. If you're thinking that, I know you don't work in the drug business. Those of you that do make your living in health care may already know I'm talking about the story of Premarin.

Premarin, an estrogen replacement product extracted from the urine of pregnant mares, and therefore "natural," was once among the most commonly prescribed drugs in the United States. I remember I once worked a grand opening for a pharmacy and panicked that we only had one bottle of 100 tablets of the most common strength of Premarin on the shelf. We weren't expecting to do more than 100 prescriptions total that day, but there was a good chance that little bottle would not hold out until closing time. Any real pharmacy would have had at least a thousand tablets in stock. It was thought of as the closest thing modern science had to a fountain of youth for women, not only treating symptoms of menopause; the hot flashes and vaginal dryness some women know all too well, but also osteoporosis, heart disease, and dementia. All while promising to help keep you looking young and sexy. Why, you'd have to be crazy **not** to want to take Premarin! And it flew off the pharmacy shelves, providing women a key weapon to maintain their health and a nice profit for Premarin's manufacturer, Wyeth. Everyone was happy.

And then the government had to step in.

The National Institutes of Health began a study in 1991 called the Women's Health Initiative in order to get a clearer picture of the effects of long term estrogen use. Eleven years later it concluded that the combination of Premarin and another hormone, Provera (medroxyprogesterone), which is used to counter the risk of endometrial cancer in women who have not undergone a hysterectomy, increased the risk of heart attack, increased the risk of stroke, increased the risk of serious blood clots and increased the risk of breast cancer in women who took it. If I remember correctly it also would set you back about $40 a month at the time. Wyeth took immediate action to get this important information out and to limit the use of Premarin and Provera to women who absolutely could not do without it. In some alternate universe that's what they did. In this universe, while government researchers were sounding the alarm over what they had found, a company by the name of DesignWrite, hired by Wyeth to get articles published in medical journals, was shopping around an article, "author to be decided" that declared hormones to be "the gold standard" for treating hot flashes. They found a doctor to claim authorship, and the article was published in The Journal of Reproductive Medicine in 2005, three years after we knew what kind of damage Premarin was doing to the women of the world. DesignWrite charged Wyeth $25,000 for the article, which evidently is the going rate for a soul these days.

Fortunately the good science eventually won, and prescriptions for Premarin, Provera, and a tablet that combined them both, Prempro, went through the floor. The fall of these meds from the lofty perch of multi-billion dollar a year blockbuster to the current accepted practice of using them in the lowest dose for the shortest term possible is credited with that ten percent drop in the breast cancer rate I mentioned earlier. One simple change in medical practice that produced an instant drop in the number of people dying in one of the most excruciating ways a person can die. And Big Pharma fought it all the way. There's part of the reason your prescription costs so much. Because the corporations that make your medicines are so desperate for every last dollar they can find that they will continue to fight for them even when they know they are killing people. I have a customer who had a mastectomy after taking Premarin for years whom I can barely look in the eye now, and I didn't ghostwrite anything. All I did was trust them.

Never again. I will never trust them again

Another Tale Of Big Pharma's Commitment To Good Science. And Women's Health.

The key to our story is this:

High doses of estrogen are known to raise the risk for blood clots that can cause heart attacks and strokes. We covered that in the last chapter.

We've known this for awhile now. Estrogen levels have been getting lower and lower in Oral Contraceptives for years, as drug companies push the envelope to see how far down they can go and maintain effectiveness. Good for them. Heart attacks and stokes tend to suck. Fourteen years ago, drugmaker Johnson & Johnson had an idea to push that envelope a little lower, at least to hear them tell it. They told the FDA their new contraceptive patch, Ortho Evra, would expose women to less estrogen than traditional birth control pills. Great. There was, of course, the formality of actually proving that women would actually be exposed to less estrogen, which as you'll remember, was known to raise the risk for blood clots that can cause heart attacks and strokes.

The studies began. They did not turn out well.

A trial finished in 1999 showed that Ortho Evra delivered about as much estrogen as an oral contraceptive that contained 76 micrograms of estrogen. Seventy-six micrograms sounds like a tiny amount, until you realize that the FDA banned birth control pills that contained more than 50 micrograms of estrogen in 1988.

Wait a minute! That's more estrogen! Which is known to raise the risk for blood clots that can cause heart attacks and strokes! Johnson & Johnson was wrong! Boy I bet they felt silly as they immediately scrapped plans for Ortho-Evra and went back to the drawing board. I mean, that's what you'd think a health care company would do.

In this case, however, the study's author applied a "correction factor" to the results of the trial. To "adjust" for the differences in the way the body would process a chemical absorbed through the skin as opposed to the GI tract. After the numbers were, ahem, "corrected," it was claimed that Ortho Evra delivered about 20 micrograms of estrogen a day. No one had mentioned the need for a "correction factor" when the study's protocol was filed with the FDA.

Problem solved.

Johnson and Johnson was so proud of the scientific breakthrough that led to the discovery of this "correction factor" that they mentioned it one time in 435 pages filed with the FDA, buried as part of a mathematical formula. Now, fancy High-falutin' scientists with PhD's and paychecks signed by Big

Pharma can come up with terms like "correction factors," but you know, simple pharmacists with Bachelors degrees and roots in the hillbilly land that is Southeastern Ohio have another term for it.

"Pulling numbers out of your ass"

The patch was approved and Johnson and Johnson told doctors Ortho Evra released 20 micrograms of estrogen into the bloodstream in 24 hours. The company now says that number is wrong, that the "correction factor" was not correct. A study done after Ortho Evra reached the market showed that women who used it had as much as twice the risk of blood clots as those who used birth control pills. Which is exactly what you would expect from being exposed to higher levels of estrogen.

Yeah, definitely pulling numbers out of your ass.

Reached for comment in an alternate universe that doesn't actually exist, Johnson & Johnson Chairman and CEO William C. Weldon said in my mind, "but it's sticky....Ortho-Evra is sticky and you can wear it"

"Just try sticking a tablet on your skin" he added in my imagination.

Thing is, Johnson & Johnson totally got this bullshit past the FDA. By massaging some numbers around, Johnson & Johnson presented an application that claimed Ortho-Evra was safer than existing contraceptive options when it was not. Underfunded, understaffed, and incompetent because it was run by political appointees who believed that government shouldn't do anything but start wars, the FDA looked at the numbers and said...."ddduuuhhhhh"

Less than two years later, the government then started a war in Iraq for no apparent reason. In a democracy you get the type of government you ask for my friends. Remember that next time you're at the ballot box.

To Prove I Am Fair And Balanced. I Will Now Share With You A Tale Of Big Pharma Looking Out For Your Financial Interest.

I feel your pain Corporate America. I know how in this dog-eat-dog ruthless cutthroat culture that is capitalism in the 21st century, a dollar wasted can mean catastrophe. Pennies must be pinched, pinched until they beg for mercy!! Unnecessary expenses are a threat to our very way of life, it says so right in the Constitution. Go ahead, read in the constitution for yourself what it says about the rights of corporations, especially the part where it defines them as artificial persons.

(psst....that was a trick. The word "corporation" never appears in the Constitution, the first three words of which are "We the people")

Corporate America, I want to do my part to help in your never-ending battle to save a buck. That's why I'm offering the Drugnazi free pharmacist salary monitoring service. Sign up for this program, and I will make sure you do not spend any more on pharmacist salaries than is absolutely necessary. I will offer helpful tips on ways to spend less on pharmacists, saving you valuable payroll dollars to use as ammunition in your battle for market share. I ask for nothing in return. I do this only because it is the right thing for you.

That's pretty messed up Drugnazi" some of you might be saying. "You can't be in charge of a program that works against your own financial self interest. This 'program' is either a sham or you have some sort of ulterior motive."

You would be right. Remember how you figured that out as I tell you how in 2003, Eli Lilly started a program to monitor that doctors were not inappropriately prescribing, and therefore wasting money on, drugs for mental illness.

Mental illness drugs like Zyprexa. Made by Lilly. I want to reiterate here that any money "wasted" on Zyprexa by doctors that don't know what they're doing goes straight into Lilly's pocket.

I think I shall also start a program to monitor the clerk at the liquor store to make sure he does not give me more scotch than I pay for.

Doctors who attracted the attention of Lilly's monitoring program got a "Dear Doctor" letter letting them know they were out of the medical mainstream. Then absolutely nothing had to happen. Because compliance in this program was entirely voluntary.

So Lilly started a program to keep an eye on doctors that used Zyprexa outside of accepted guidelines. Good for them. I wonder, though, if the official FDA approved indications for Zyprexa would be considered a guideline? Because in 2009, Lilly paid over $1.4 billion dollars to settle claims it marketed Zyprexa for uses not approved by the FDA, like the treatment of dementia in the elderly. After Lilly engaged in conduct in which they admitted no guilt but cost them almost a billion and a half dollars, it was shown that elderly patients suffering from dementia that were given Zyprexa-like drugs were more likely to die than a placebo group. Maybe Lilly will send itself a letter. Of course compliance is voluntary.

You might think Lilly monitoring doctors to make sure doctors don't put money in Lilly's pocket is a "funny in a stupid way" kind of story, and it is, but there is also a dash of "scary in an evil way" spice to this. The program also monitored patients, specifically whether they were having prescriptions refilled, and notified their doctor if they were not.

So.....if a person decides they would rather deal with their mental health problems instead of dealing with the weight gain, high cholesterol and high blood sugar levels Zyprexa can cause, Lilly, out of only concern for the patient mind you, would report that person to the proper health care authorities. And you lose another bit of your personal sovereignty to help out the bottom line of a corporation whose profits in 2009 worked out to be around $494,000 an hour. Nothing like living in the land of the free.

I think I hear voices in my head...........

Wow, This Is Getting Depressing, I'm Going To Lighten The Mood With A Workplace Story.

The upside down ointment cap was the last straw. "THIS TUBE IS DEFECTIVE!" screamed the lunatic. "I WANT MY MONEY BACK!!"

The Pharmacy Manager calmly showed the lunatic that the defect was that he was trying to put the cap on, yes, upside down. The lunatic wouldn't budge. He wasn't leaving until he got a new tube. I knew caving in a few months ago when he demanded a refund for a three-quarters empty bottle of eye drops because "he wasn't satisfied with the product" would only lead to trouble. The Pharmacy Manager wouldn't listen to me then. Now I was the only one who could bail her out. As the lunatic walked out the door with his new ointment tube, she said "I will buy a 12 pack of beer for anyone who can run that man off."

Everyone in the pharmacy knew who "anyone" was. This was a job for The Drugnazi, and I understood the parameters of the mission, should I choose to accept it. It was to be a clandestine operation. Should any part of it become public, those who sent me in would deny all knowledge of it or me. This tape will self-destruct in 15 seconds.

I also knew what I was up against. I had waited on the lunatic for many months and had never once acted like I had appreciated his business in any way, yet he kept coming back. That kind of thing happens when you keep giving them free prescriptions. This would not be easy. But there was free beer. I set my terms.

"You're not talking Milwaukee's Best are you?"

"Anything in the store."

"I'm in"

I started with the "out of stock" trick. Totally untraceable. How many pharmacies have ever really run out of Vicodin? None that want to stay in business, as generic Vicodin tablets are usually the most profitable thing a pharmacy carries, but that's exactly what happened the next two times the lunatic came to the counter.

This was coupled with the "exaggerated order time" maneuver. It takes a week to order Vicodin. When you're a lunatic that is.

Closely related to this is "exaggerated fill time" When there's a beer bounty on your head, it takes an hour to fill your prescription. Then when you come back in an hour it's not quite done.

At this point, regular customers of most chain drugstores may be saying to themselves, "You mean there are places where this type of thing would be considered unusual?"

Even with all this, I still needed a bit of luck. The lunatic called at 5 minutes to closing one night and wanted me to stay late. That usually doesn't happen even when I like you, and there's no chance when you're a half empty ointment tube returning lunatic. The next day another pharmacy called to transfer "all his prescriptions." I emptied out his profile and sent it over, and that night happily cracked open an imported Pale Ale.

Of course I suppose I could have bought my own beer when all this started, but beer tastes better when you earn it.

Mission Accomplished.

More Reasons Your Prescription Can Cost So Much. Sometimes Drug Companies Charge You Through The Nose For Nothing But A Different Name

So by now you're familiar with the "just different enough to get a new patient" tactic Big Pharma employs with regularity to shore up their bottom line, and you may think whoever thought of that little isomer trick was one clever little capitalist. You'd be right. You may also admire whoever first thought of the "ER" trick, charging more money for a longer lasting version of the exact same drug. Draining your wallet isn't just a job for the science folks though. There are times when all you need is a gift for marketing and a different label. Since the beginning of my pharmacy career, I've been keeping an eye out for the most pointless, inane, rip-off piece of crap peddled by Big Pharma. There has never been a shortage of contenders, and I can't think of a better way to spend part of my day right now than by going over a few. That's what I do. I'm the Drugnazi.

For your consideration:

Niravam- An orally disintegrating form of alprazolam, an anti-anxiety med available for years as Xanax and as a cheap as dirt generic. Not only will Niravam cost you more than 5 times the price of generic alprazolam, but alprazolam tablets are among the smallest you're gonna find, making the benefit of an orally disintegrating version a little dubious. But, I suppose there might be one or two people out there a bit too life challenged to swallow a tablet the size of a grain of rice. (Price comparison from drugstore.com)

Bidil- A combination of isosorbide dinitrate and hydralazine, two meds that have been on the market for years and are also cheap as dirt. Bidil combines the two old meds into one tablet, and then markets itself to African-Americans as a race specific remedy for heart failure. Of course there's no reason you can't prescribe the two drugs separately and save money, but hey, maybe it is easier for people to just swallow one tablet, and at least there is research to support the claim this combination of meds is more effective for black folks.

Moving up a level on the rip off scale we have:

Sarafem- The exact same thing as Prozac. The exact, same, thing. Except it comes in a different box so someone snooping in your medicine cabinet will just see that you're PMSing and not clinically depressed.

Proquin XR- A pointless version of extended release ciprofloxacin, an antibiotic. The labeling says to take it with food, so the manufacturer of

Proquin XR can claim it causes less stomach upset when taken as directed than the other extended release version of ciprofloxacin on the market, Cipro XR.

There's no way it can get worse than the med you are about to meet though, unless Big Pharma starts to make products that are actually less effective and more expensive than what they're designed to replace. Crap. Probably just gave them an idea. Anyway..... drum roll please.............

Introducing Pexeva. Brand name for paroxetine mesylate.

Paroxetine is already sold under the brand name Paxil. Paxil lost it's patent a few years back, and I've already discussed Paxil CR, itself a contender for most useless piece of drug crap ever. Pexeva though, is not a continuous release version of paroxetine. It doesn't come in a different package telling you it's for a different indication. It's not orally disintegrating. The maker of Pexeva, JDS Pharmaceuticals, has made it just different enough from Paxil (it is a different salt form, mesylate vs. HCl) that a pharmacist cannot substitute one for the other. Then they don't even respect your intelligence enough to try and bullshit you into thinking that makes any difference whatsoever in the two meds. They just want you to buy Pexeva, and pay 69% more for it than you would for generic paroxetine, (Price comparison from Consumer Reports)

Which leads to the question, why would any doctor ever write a prescription for Pexeva?

Because they're a dumbass, that's why. And if a Pexeva prescription is ever handed to you, tell your doctor I said so.

Speaking Of Pexeva, Every Once In Awhile I Can Win One.

Most of the time I never hear back from people once I dispense advice, and when I do, any reaction I get will more often than not be skepticism. More times than you might imagine, when a person asks me a question, what they are looking for isn't an answer so much as a debate. When this happens I think a lot about chicken fat. One day when I was in college me and a group of friends were trading stories about who had the worst job when we were in high school. The winner had to go into a giant vat at a slaughterhouse where live chickens had been dropped in boiling water all day long and clean out a shift's worth of congealed fat from the walls. We all agreed back then that was pretty disgusting, but now that I think about it, I bet chicken fat removers are appreciated by the people who show up to a nice clean vat every morning. Appreciated, wanted even. Which is more than I get when I try to tell you there's a good chance a $20 dollar box of Prilosec OTC will work as well as your $173 Nexium prescription. Imagine my surprise then, when this showed up one day in my mailbox:

> I just wanted to thank you immensely for telling me about idiotic doctors who give Pexeva prescriptions instead of paroxetine. My husband was diagnosed as bipolar about a year ago. We have been in terrible financial condition, in large part to his inability to work because of his mental issues. After years of discussion, I finally got him to see a doctor about it. He was diagnosed using the same damn checklist I found online years before and the doctor prescribed Pexeva. It was like a miracle -- he was under control for the first time in a long time. The only problem was that his prescription cost about $200 a month (he's uninsured), and it was very hard to scrape the money together to pay for it.
>   Our dumbass doctor didn't believe there was a generic Pexeva (amazing!!) Incredibly, it took some arm-twisting to get the damn paroxetine prescription from him, but we got it. $4 freaking dollars a month at any Wal-Mart or Kroger's; hell of a difference from $200 a month. Honestly, we can now pay the electric bill thanks to you!!!

If things like this happened more often, I might reconsider my future in the chicken-fat removal business. Unfortunately, they don't. Most days are more like this, which is why I think a lot about starting a business that would remove chicken fat from wherever it might accumulate:

I had the brainstorm of brainstorms when I saw the Coors Light truck. The Coors Light truck always filled me with a sense of desperation, appearing as it does in front of the store on Friday mornings. Fridays were my twelve hour days you see, and seeing that truck at the beginning of a twelve hour shift each and every week became a bit Pavlovian.

This day, however, the Coors Light truck triggered my brainstorm. I decided I would learn Arabic. Surely people that speak Arabic have no trouble getting decent paying jobs at the CIA, especially people who can prove without much effort they've never been to a Taliban training camp. My God, I could escape my job once and for all while at the same time learning lots and lots of secrets. I love secrets. I'd get a regular lunch break too and maybe even find Osama Bin Laden.

I walked in the door and the clerk manning the front register asked me what it means when your poop is blue-green and I crashed back into reality. I asked the first person to come to the counter whether we had filled prescriptions for him before or if this would be the first time.

"Both" he said. I didn't ask. I just got their information. I have learned that anything other than an unqualified "yes" means "get all my information."

The first fax of the day was from my employer's technical support department. The store manager had e-mailed them the night before that our phones were not working, and the fax said they were trying to call about his email but couldn't get through because the phones didn't seem to be working. My employer's decision to fix the phones with used parts salvaged from other phone systems the month before was really paying off in terms of time saved and increased business opportunities.

We settled into our regular prescription filling routine, which was made far more pleasant by the fact there were no phones. For some reason I started telling my Supertech about the days before real-time insurance claims. "We had this thing like a giant 8-track player, and you would put this huge-ass tape into it, then the computer would put all your Medicaid claims for the week on it. Took about half an hour. Then you sent it into the corporate office and like a month later you'd get this printout with all the rejects you were supposed to fix."

I looked up and the hottest chick in the world was staring right at me. Nothing like showing the ladies how much of an old fart you are. I am one smooth operator. Although later on I'm pretty sure a customer told me she loved me. She said it as she was leaving, kinda like you would to your husband, without thinking about it. I decided I'll take my affection where I can get it.

A person asked where the bathroom was, as they needed to wash their hands because some hand sanitizer had spilled on them.

My other technician for the day was a rent-a-tech from another location in my employer's chain and he was...how do I put this?...terrible. I overheard him trying to deal with a customer upset with the amount of his insurance co-pay. "THIS IS A CROCK OF SHIT!!" I heard the customer say, and my heart leapt for joy. It's not often these opportunities present themselves. I walked over and relieved the rent-a-tech of his cashier duties.

"It will be just as much a crock of shit no matter where you go sir. Now, do you want to watch your language or do you want to go somewhere else?" Because anyone who knows me knows that I'm all about keeping the language clean.

The phone rang a few minutes later and startled us all. "Do you carry eyelash glue?" The man asked, and I chose to frame the experience in a positive light. Not that someone couldn't listen to the store's voicemail system and therefore ended up talking to the pharmacy when they shouldn't have, but that I had the chance to learn that people evidently put glue on their eyelashes for some reason. I bet that piece of knowledge will come in handy sometime when I least expect it.

The next call was pharmacy related. "My dad takes warfarin and this Pepto bottle says to ask your doctor before mixing it with warfarin. So I should just give him half as much, right?" I have no idea how the half-dose idea got into that woman's head and even though I talked her out of it, I still feared for her father's life.

Around the time we discovered the rent-a-tech sold the wrong prescription to a customer, a large group of men came in and started making noises that sounded something like "ahut a alubba eght ahloo" over and over again. One of them started waving around a blood sugar monitor and making noises that sounded a little different, almost familiar. He expected me to respond to the noise.

I did, by saying, "I'm sorry, I don't understand" This made the entire group repeat the noise louder. This went on for a good two or three minutes before I saw a customer walking away from the counter with his prescription for Keflex, an antibiotic related to penicillin. Rent-a-tech had decided to ignore the tag that said "PENICILLIN ALLERGY" I had placed inside the bag and I had to almost tackle the customer as they walked away. My reward when I returned was a now angry group of noisemakers.

"Is this.....universal? I could buy in Iraq?" One of them finally said. I simultaneously wondered why in the hell this guy wasn't doing the talking in the first place and realized what language they were speaking.

Arabic. I still haven't decided whether this was a sign from Karma that I should go for my dream or a dire warning that she was not to be fucked with.

I washed away the day with a twelve pack of Coors Light. It seemed appropriate.

Actually I Wouldn't Have To Start That Chicken Fat Removal Business If I Could Just Learn How To Eat Grass.

I almost wrote the Unabomber once. I wanted to learn from him, not how to make bombs, blow stuff up and not get caught for years, but how he managed to live out there in that little cabin of his in the middle of nowhere, Montana, and not starve to death. If you work in retail pharmacy and tell me you have never fantasized about putting as much distance as possible between you and every other human on the planet, I know you're lying. Consider that I never particularly cared for humans in the first place, and you can see why if you take out the violence, Ted Kaczynski was living the life of my dreams.

Unfortunately I have to eat, and the skills I have that would enable me to live off the land are very close to zero, which led me to ponder picking the brain of the Unabomber. I figured he probably didn't have much to do these days, but in the end, I decided it's probably a good idea to try to avoid things that get you on lists compiled by federal law enforcement. So the idea went dormant, along with my plans for becoming a chess grandmaster, learning the bass guitar, and writing a Broadway musical based on the life of Iggy Pop. Until one day that is, when I saw a herd of cows.

"Goddamn cows" I said to myself as I drove along, consumed with jealousy as I went past them on the way to work. Even knowing I would be slaughtered in the end, I would totally trade their life of leisurely standing around in a field all day for mine of listening to the great unwashed masses sing the praises of stool softeners. Then I realized. The cows were standing around all day.....eating grass. Not only eating grass mind you, but meeting all their energy and nutritional needs while doing so. Grass is everywhere. If I could unlock the cow's secret. I could live anywhere. I could live.....in a cabin....in the middle of nowhere.

To those of you who say cows don't have much in the way of energy needs, I would submit the buffalo, also an eater of plants, or the antelope. Of course I would have to keep the historical human ability to keep predators at bay, which is the weak point of most herbivores, but we put a man on the moon for Chrissakes, are you telling me we can't figure out how to digest a friggin plant? If the chlorophyll turned me green, I'd still be OK with that.

That day I saw the future, or at least the key to my future liberation, and it is grass. At least until they start charging for air.

I'm Not Bitter About The Lack Of A Little Plastic Stunt Motorcycle Christmas. Really, I'm Not

You know, for someone who professes to love us all, you'd think that maybe the thought our time could be worth a little something might enter Jesus' skull once or twice. That maybe Jesus could tell us, "You know, there's no need to go all out for my birthday. Really. Me and my Dad, the all knowing, omnipotent creator of universes known and unknown, the Deity that can part seas with his breath, move mountains with his pinky and knows the exact number of hairs on your head, I'm sure we'll come up with something. Don't put yourself out just on my account."

"And there is really no need to invent The Clapper to sell in the season of my special day. You work too hard for your money."

That's what my Uncle Harold would say. Uncle Harold always insisted we never make a big deal about his birthday, because that was just the kind of guy Harold was. Unlike this prick Jesus who pretty much ruined my whole week last year with this Christmas shit.

And by whole week I mean entire month of December. And part of November as well. Traffic gets backed up because of a goddamn parade. People everywhere I want to shop. A big pile of pine trees right where I normally park my car at work. All because this savior of mankind lets it go straight to his head.

I got news for you Jesus. I once saved the life of a mouse we found in the backroom of the store. That's right. Instead of killing it, I captured the little guy and let him loose in the woods in back of the mall. And I don't expect the mouse to buy shit every year for my birthday either. I think maybe I could teach you a thing or two about humility Mr. Son of God.

The sad thing is it's not just me that gets screwed. The entire goddamn planet has to put their lives on hold just for Jesus every year. Fuck it makes me so mad. I got over birthdays when I was like 9, and Jesus still gets all giddy like a girl after 2000 of them? Give me a break.

Buddhism looks better every day. No wonder there are so many Buddhists.

Totally Not Bitter.

If I Were Rudolph The Reindeer, I Would Have Told Santa To Go Fuck Himself.

I would have been like. "You bastards have given me shit my whole life and NOW you want me to bail you out?? You can kiss my reindeer ass"

Then I would have been like "You know, while I was excluded and ostracized all those years, I worked on a few reindeer games of my own, since you would never let me play any of yours" There would be a crazy look in my eye.

Then I would take off and fly around in circles while Dancer and Prancer and the rest of those asswipes sat grounded with all the undeliverable toys on the shipping dock. Every once in awhile I would swoop down and kick them in the head or maybe bite them in the back while yelling "WHAT CHA THINK OF MY NOSE NOW MUTHA FUCKER?? TELL ME WHAT YOU THINK OF MY NOSE!!!!!"

I guess that wouldn't be a good way to mark Jesus' birthday though. I mean, Jesus would never punish you years after the fact for being a bad person.

Not Warped Either.

He kept up appearances for the children. That is the epitaph to remember Frosty by always. Frosty loved the children.

Frosty knew the sun was hot that day. He knew his fate. But Frosty chose to spend what remained of his time living, not dying. He took his broomstick and he ran here and there, around the square, leading the nation's children into a rebellion not of street gangs, violent crime, teenage pregnancy or any of the other social ills that plague our youth, but a rebellion of joy.

He even paused for a moment when the town square's traffic cop called for him to stop, for Frosty was at his core a good and decent soul.

Frosty is gone now, a victim of seasonal change and global warming. Most of his corpse is scattered in the vast nothingness of this planet's oceans, some of it refroze and may be trapped glacially for millennia, some is locked underground, and some may be carrying away the sewage of the fetid masses of humanity, but the magical moment he gave our children will never die. Which is why I hope.... no, which is why I know, that someday Frosty will know the magic that is a trip over Yosemite falls.

I think I may have just peed out a piece of Frosty.

There Is One Christmas Tradition I Hold Dear However

Back Door Santa. To me, Christmas is all about the Back Door Santa.

I suppose I should probably explain.

Back in the carefree days when presidents struggled to define the word "is" and not the word "torture," I found an old vinyl copy of *A Very Special Christmas*, an album put together to benefit a charity of some sort, at my favorite thrift shop. It was like a little time capsule of the popular music scene of the late 80's. Bruce Springsteen was there, along with Sting, RUN-D.M.C. and Whitney Houston among others. I once had a dream about Whitney Houston, whom I at one time thought was the most beautiful woman in the world. In my dream I emerged from a locker room to take part in a track meet. As I took the field, the electricity amongst the crowd was overwhelming, as Whitney Houston was there. You see, in my dream, before her singing career and years of drug-fueled creatively inactive notoriety, Whitney had been a star of track and field, and this event was to be the start of her comeback. Whitney was wearing a black fishnet, spandexy thing that was not flattering to the pounds she'd picked up over the years. During the race, Whitney and I were lapped by the eventual winner, even though we were competing in the 100 yard dash. I finished the event in what seemed like around three hours in next to last place, ahead of only Whitney Houston.

Other than my college crush on her, I have no idea what this whole episode says about my subconscious mind. Maybe I should lay off the melatonin.

Back to the record though, that little round portal into the world of my youth. You couldn't have a benefit album back then without U2. I miss Bono. I admit I only bought a copy of *War*, unheard, when I was in junior high because I thought *Sunday Bloody Sunday* was one of the coolest song titles ever. It did turn out to be a pretty cool song, but not for the reasons the little 13 year old Beavis was thinking. *Bloody Sunday*, for those of you who don't know, was written about a day when the British military shot 27 protesters in the city of Derry, Northern Ireland. Thirteen died. Seven children. Tonight we can be as one Bono sang. Everyone, on both sides, can agree this never should have happened. Heavy stuff. Exactly the kind of stuff a child redneck needed to hear.

But it didn't end there. Around the time I would have seen my first black person, I got hit with *Pride (In The Name of Love)* Of course I didn't understand when Bono sang how they took a man's life but not his pride. But the obvious power and passion with which those words were delivered made me want to learn. It's a good thing for child rednecks to want to learn. And the more I learned the more I cherished those words. Those words that were a rock thrown against the wall of injustice that was built, guarded, and made unchangeable by the powerful and privileged. Fine. They can keep it. There are things that are more important, even at the expense of your life. They never took Dr. King's pride.

But it didn't end there. In college the child redneck caught *Rattle and Hum,* the flick, as a Saturday midnight movie, and afterwards the child redneck decided not to sell his soul to the ROTC for college money. "No more!" chanted Bono. And there would be no more. Jesus, Mary and Joseph I will never forget the atmosphere in that theater as the movie ended. I would not be in the ROTC, I would be in an army of 20 year olds who were soon to be unleashed on the world who would put up with no more. We were young, we were energy, and Goddammit, things were gonna change.

I soon thereafter sold my soul to retail pharmacy and started to meekly fill prescriptions. U2 soon thereafter released *Achtung Baby,* a fine but noticeably meeker record.

My next U2 crowd experience came in Los Angeles almost 12 years later. I looked around and saw the army of the young and impassioned had become the sportcoat wearing paunchy and balding, waving to their friends on the other side of the arena while using their cellphone. George W. Bush was president, and he was about to show the nation the glory of invading a country that did not attack us. The music had been neutered. I think that night was the first time I felt old. Maybe the next generation.....

None of that was going through my head the first time I saw *A Very Special Christmas* however. I bought it for only one reason, the prospect of hearing Jon Bon Jovi sing a song called *Back Door Santa.* The thought of Jon Bon Jovi as a Back Door Santa was frighteningly alluring.

Jon did not disappoint. The tune is delightfully horrible. It's an old Blues number redone in 80's hairband excess, right down to the piped-in fake crowd noise. Every time I hear the opening power keyboard riff, I never fail to laugh non-stop for a good four minutes. It's unintentionally hilarious, which is the worst way to suck.....if you're a band. Jon sounds like he's taking himself so seriously in the song, I honestly wonder if he knew how the words "Back Door Santa" could be interpreted, and that at the time he totally looked like a girl.

At any rate, *Back Door Santa* became a holiday tradition around the Drugnazi household. It started with a girlfriend who would only consent to listen to the song one time between Thanksgiving and Christmas. Naturally, I would try to pick the time that would produce maximum annoyance, which is probably part of the reason she is now an ex-girlfriend. She's long gone, but the tradition of the once-annual playing of *Back Door Santa* remains. Yes, I could listen to *Back Door Santa* whenever I want to now, but that would be like eating turkey every day. The holidays should stand for something dammit.

I miss Bono. All the more so because he's still around.

A Mystery Present Doesn't Help Me With My Christmas Issues.

It happens every year. Some mystery customer comes in when I'm not working and drops off little presents for the pharmacy staff. I don't mean that the customer is trying to be mysterious, I mean that even after seeing the name on the tag, I wouldn't know who this customer is if they came up and bit me on the nads. I mean, I guess it's a nice gesture and all, but honestly, I've said for years the best way to show your gratitude for me doing my job is by shutting up, taking your stuff, and getting away from the counter as soon as possible. Seriously. I will appreciate your quick exit more than anything you can do or say.

Anyway, this year's present from the mystery customer was a manicure set. Wait. Maybe this wasn't a nice gesture at all. Maybe my hands so disgust this person that they have been moved to try to relieve themselves of beholding their grotesqueness ever again. Could it be that part of me is.......unattractive? Suddenly I was intrigued by the manicure set and the possibility of becoming even hotter.

Except that I don't know what half the things in the manicure set are. There's like three sets of nail clippers, which is seven short of one for each of my nails, a set of tweezers, a utensil I had never owned until that day, a little pair of scissors, a nail file that totally doesn't look like a nail file, and then this group of unidentifiables:

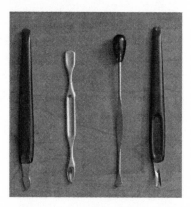

I am honest to God stumped. The thing on the left has an angled edge like some sort of knife. Cuticle pusher backer? Could the fact I'm not pushing back my cuticles be the reason I'm not getting laid at the moment?

If the thing second from the left were a little bigger, it might be the type of object you use to dig out some caviar to spread on your Ritz cracker or whatever it is you eat caviar on. Maybe with the economy being the way it is, the average caviar portion size has gone way down. Wait. This is part of a manicure set, so caviar server doesn't make any sense. I bet you might be able to use it to actually pry one of your fingernails off though. Is that some sort of new fad among the kids nowdays maybe?

My best guess for the third thing is an earwax digger. Except it kinda tickles when I gently probe my ear canal with it. Maybe it's some sort of ear dildo.

Dammit. I can't hear anything all the sudden. I should probably go to the ER when I'm done writing this.

I'm thinking the last thing is a nose picker. See how the end of it is like a two-pronged fork? Bet you could totally spear a booger with this. Perhaps that is the civilized way to clear your nasal passageways in high society. A finger does seem sort of barbaric.

So anyway, any help you guys could give me here would be appreciated. If you have any clues, feel free to zap them to me at drugmonkeyrph@gmail.com. With your assistance, I may end this year hotter than I began it. Or at least avoid large hospital bills.

Thanks in advance.

OK, Since I Don't Think The Little Plastic Stunt Motorcycle Is Ever Gonna Happen, I've Finally Decided What I Want For Christmas.

I don't shop anywhere near where I work. I never have. I've split my career between the ghetto and the bastions of some of the world's most affluent people and I don't like to hang around either place for any longer than I have to. A guy's gotta eat though, and when that guy's too lazy and organizationally inept to pack his own food, that means he gets to spend his lunch time blending in with what passes for the elite in our society. Getting mistaken for one of them when all I want is a sandwich or something.

I also get to see the interaction of classes in our society, as even the most snobby of snobby shopping centers cannot function without hiring people to take care of the garbage, fix the potholes in the parking lot, or paint the wall across from Macy's. Of course when I say "interaction of classes in our society" what I mean is the total lack thereof, as the janitors, the maintenance people, and the painters have all been trained to be nearly invisible so as to not disturb the people with the money. I see one woman almost every day with a broom and a dustpan walking the grounds, sweeping up cigarette butts and other little bits of miscellaneous trash. She's a little part of my life almost every working day, and she's almost as good at averting her eyes from the customers as she is at keeping the grounds butt-free. Just once I'd like to give her a little smile and a hello, but short of tackling her I don't think it's gonna happen. She's been trained to be invisible. The only hellos I ever get are from the affluent assholes.

For Christmas I would like that woman to not expect to be invisible. I'd like to look her in the eye and smile and say hi, like you would think would happen between any two people in a civilized society. To mark the holiday, I want her to not turn her head. To not feel as if that's what's expected of her. That's pretty much the whole of my list this year. I'm not into tackling anyone though, so I'll settle for her having a good holiday in whatever world it's acceptable for her to be seen.

I guess you should have a good holiday too.

I Fought The Mall And The Mall Won. She Fought The Mall And Kicked Its Ass.

So, yes, I work at a mall. I am not proud of this. As a matter of fact, it grates my ass from the moment I pull into the mall and see that goddamn water fountain of theirs next to the street. I live in an area of chronic water shortage, where an average person can fight for years to put in a second bathroom and the mall thinks it's a great thing to shoot water around for the hell of it all day long. Someday I'm gonna put so much dish soap in that water fountain it will be both ruined and squeaky clean for at least 20 years.

It's more than water waste that puts the burr up my butt though. The mall as an institution is a monument to the cheap crap made in China sell your soul to corporate control complex that rules us. Your definition of what is beautiful comes from Victoria's Secret. Your good taste from the Pottery Barn. Your culture from the cineplex down at the south end. And if your money comes from the mall, God have mercy on your soul, because you will be broken before a check is ever issued. Take a good look at the people behind the counter at your favorite store at the mall my friends. They're either high school kids or they are broken.

And if any of this starts to bother you, that's when you come down to the north end of the mall and see me. To get the chemicals that will make you forget all about it. Unless you're me. They don't sell my brand of scotch at the mall.

The lady at the pizza place seemed to be an exception though. I could never quite put my finger on it, but she definitely wasn't broken. Her smile always seemed so........real. It was evident that she lived within the mall culture but was not of it. I sensed something. I totally sensed something, but could never quite tell what it was.

Until one day when I read in the local alterna-weekly about the lady who used to work at the pizza place's CD release party. I went. I have no friends mind you, and I hate going to places by myself. But I went because I desperately wanted her to be good. I wanted so much for the mall to finally lose a round.

The mall lost a round that night my friends. I am a music snob, and as such I would be unable to tell you she was good if she was not. She made my ears happy for a little over an hour that night, and a little bit of my soul happy for a good deal longer than that. Because the mall lost one, and I didn't have to   break out the dish soap. It's not making contact with the lady who sweeps up the cigarette butts, but it'll make for an OK Christmas this year.

In your face mall

Just Another Random Workday

Five minutes after opening Supertech comes waltzing in and I just couldn't do it. It was witty maybe the first 25 times I said it, but the horse was just so dead that I would be beating. I sat in silence for maybe 30 seconds. Struggling. "Don't say it." I thought to myself. "Distract yourself with thoughts of scotch and such."

"I know, nice of me to join you." Supertech blurted out as she put on her lab coat. We're getting to know each other too well I fear. I need some new material, and she needs to stop coming in late.

First words out of the first customer of the day: "Three years ago I had all my teeth." My hopes for the day soared. How on earth can any day that starts with those words be a bad one?

I settled into the Friday double-V routine. Viagra and Vicodin. I have Friday regulars for each. One of my Viagra regulars came in with his wife. I understood his need for the V. Supertech rings him up and wifey explodes.

"WHAT??????!!!!!! WE'RE NOT PAYING THAT.....FOR THIS??? THERE IS NO WAY ON EARTH HONEY!!!!"

Supertech did what she usually does in price-complaint situations. Checks to see what they paid last time. She broke the news to wifey.

"YOU HAVE GOT TO BE KIDDING ME!!!!! FOR THIS????????"

I seriously think I saw the dude shrinking as he stood there next to his wife as she screamed that his intimate encounters were not worth $150 a month. I was distracted by the sound of the Red Hot Chili Peppers *Under The Bridge* wafting from the in-store radio system. I chuckled at the thought of a song about shooting heroin being played in the land of the squares where I now work. Later I hoped the shrunken dude didn't think I was chuckling at him. Uptight rich white people unwittingly listening to heroin music is way funnier than a guy who can't get it up.

Then the great bag crisis hit. It had been coming for some time.

My employer has a system that involves putting finished prescriptions and their paperwork in clear plastic bags to be hung up to await the customer's arrival. Nothing fancy mind you, just a bag with a snap top closure. We'd been running low for awhile and the pharmacy manager placed an order for more foolishly thinking that is how we would get more. It's not that simple with my employer, who has decided the bags are expensive. There are procedures to be followed. District Managers to get involved. "I"s to be dotted and "T"s to be crossed. We'd been going through the hoops for a month and now....there were no bags. I sent Supertech to the pickup wall to see if any customers had prescriptions in more than one bag. I imagined that my store's enforced bag frugality would be the one event that returned our company to profitability this quarter and felt good about my service to the corporation.

Is anyone else bummed out about how there is almost no classical music on the radio anymore? Back in the day you could count on National Public Radio to give you a fix in the afternoon or late at night, but then they discovered that more news = more dollars during pledge drives. So now in addition to the edition that comes out every morning and the consideration we give all things in the late afternoon, we're on point and listening to the world and importing news from the BBC and breathing fresh air, which used to be a show about the arts, and whoever decided to let the nails screeching on a chalkboard that is Diane Rhem's voice to ever be broadcast on the radio should be waterboarded.

Where was I going with this? Oh...the classical music. I found a great way around this problem. Anytime I want to hear some classical music I just call the big chain drugstore on the other side of town, and I am treated to a good 20 minutes or so before a clerk picks up and puts me back on hold to talk to the pharmacist.

And by 20 minutes I mean half an hour.

Ten minutes into this I took a prescription from a doctor's office bimbo. Tussionex suspension, two teaspoonfuls twice a day. Exactly twice the maximum recommended daily dose of two teaspoons in 24 hours. I asked if the kindly bimbo might double check the directions with the doctor. Because I am a goddamn Superpharmacist and you don't get this shit past me.

The least of your problems if you take twice the recommended dose of a narcotic cough syrup like Tussionex would be some opioid-induced constipation. As I was waiting for the return of the bimbo a customer coincidentally asked if there was something he could take to get his pipes flowing again while he took his Vicodin. Remember it was double-V Friday.

"Why don't you use some Senokot. You can find it down aisle 5"

"Well what do you recommend?"

Bimbo called back. "The doctor said to change the Tussionex to one to two teaspoons every four to six hours"

"So...four teaspoons a day was twice the maximum dose...and you solve the problem by prescribing up to twelve teaspoonfuls a day?"

With those words I seemed to enter some sort of suspension of the time-space continuum. I felt myself rise, above the earth and towards the clouds, slipping free of the bonds that bind us to this planet, much the way I bet a daredevil must feel the moment his motorcycle becomes airborne.

I soon crashed. "I'll just phone it in somewhere else!!" Bimbo said, and my license jumped for joy. Pharmacy students take heed. Your head is being filled with clinical situations, pharmacokinetic equations and such, but the times you will actually be making a difference in the real world of retail will more often than not just involve grade school arithmetic and letting people know you just made a recommendation.

I hung up the phone and heard a ghostly laugh. I knew it was the laugh of the daredevil, but I knew not why, or if I could ever break the curse of the little plastic stunt motorcycle that haunted my life.

I ran out of bags two more times before my store manager brought up a case from the back. The sticker on the box showed they had been sitting back there for 2 years. My store manager was the most competent person I had ever seen in my organization. He was new and I suspected if he didn't cut it out he would soon be fired.

I also wonder if I'll have all my teeth in three years. I'm going to go floss now.

Upon Further Reflection, I Wonder If My Thoughts Didn't Somehow Kill That Daredevil.

I mean, seriously, the first time I thought about that motorcycle in years and he died the next day. I'm sensing there may be some big-time bad karma involved with that motorcycle that my Mom was hip to.

I'm going to slowly back away from the topic of the little plastic stunt motorcycle and never mention it again. I'm not going against Karma and I learned long ago not to go against my Mom. My Mom isn't a pharmacist, or a doctor, or nuclear engineer or rocket scientist, although she most certainly could have been. She taught me to read before I ever set foot in a classroom and I used that skill to make fun of the other illiterate kindergarten kids. I'll always be grateful to her for allowing me to discover the great self-satisfaction that comes from making other people feel bad about themselves. The most important lesson she ever taught me though, came from a box of vinyl records.

Nothing but good comes from vinyl records. Remember that.

My Mom gave them to me when I got my turntable, probably just glad to get rid of them, but what a gold mine. Time in a box from the pop crooner era of the early 50's. Lots of songs by guys who sang them wearing tuxedos, drinking martinis, and always with a proper band behind them. Trombones, clarinets.....but absolutely no Elvis Presley.

I asked Mom about this. "Oh I didn't like him" she said, and I gained valuable insight into the youth of my mother. I was the child of a nerd. Who didn't like Elvis in the 50's?

I also noticed how the collection abruptly ended around the time my parents got married. Normal enough I suppose. People grow up and move on and the music isn't nearly as important as it used to be when there's a family to raise. Then I saw the orange label. Obviously out of place amongst the drab dullness of the others. The font, the coloring....it was immediately obvious this disc was from another era.

Helen Reddy's *I Am Woman*, sitting right there next to Dean Martin. I started thinking about what could have possibly driven Mom to set foot in a record store 20 years after she had last been in one, and despite my absolute lifelong certainty that I knew it all and my head was secure, insight found a way to sneak in.

It seeped in actually. Slowly. In fits and starts like the gradual certainty of the change of seasons. Even though by early 2008 I was among the most manic of Obamamaniacs, by the time Mom told me she was donating to

49

Hillary Clinton's presidential campaign right in the thick of a primary fight that was threatening to tear apart the Democratic Party, I understood. More than I ever let on, I understood that it wasn't that long ago that if you had both a brain and a vagina, pretty much your only hope was to pass some of that gray matter through the birth canal and hope HE would be able to make some use of it. Mom worked as a secretary for awhile 'till she found herself a man and started breeding. She's also one of very few people I'll concede is smarter than myself.

So I also understand now why she cried when I got my sorry ass through college. I thought it was kinda weird at the time, but that orange record was the catalyst to a lot of insight.

Hillary was historic. More than I ever let on while I was rooting for Barack Obama. It'll happen Mom.

And when it does it won't be because she married well.

Speaking Of That Hard Fought Democratic Primary Race of 2008, Can't You Just Totally See This Happening?

The scene, inside an airplane somewhere between Iowa and New Hampshire, the night of January 3rd, 2008. Hillary Clinton has just finished 3rd in the Iowa presidential caucus, meaning the once all-but-certain Democratic nominee is now in the fight of her political life. All is silent on the plane, except for the laughter of Bill Clinton as he chats with a campaign aide, heard above the sound of jet engines:

Bill Clinton: "......oh man...what a week. I almost forgot how much I liked the mayor of Davenport. It was good to reconnect.....kinda wish I had made him Secretary of Agriculture now like I promised I was going to. Lots of good memories...." He knocks back the last of a scotch and soda.

Campaign Aide: "Remember when we went through.....where was it? Des Moines or Cedar Rapids? At that rally in '96 and that chick lifted her shirt and had "Bob Dole can suck these" written across her boobs? That's about all Mr. Viagra could have done with that woman."

Bill and the campaign aide again burst out in inappropriately loud drunken laughter. The rest of the plane is deathly silent. Hillary Clinton stares out of the window and snaps a pen in half.

Bill walks to the back of the plane and returns minutes later with two handfuls of food and drink. After settling into his seat he looks over at Hillary.

"Doughnut?" He asks.

Hillary lunges across the aisle and grabs Bill by the testicles.

"I SWEAR TO GOD IF YOU DO NOT SHUT UP RIGHT NOW YOU WILL NEVER USE THESE AGAIN!!!!!!"

The tensest of all silences now engulfs the cabin. Hillary releases her death grip after about 30 seconds. Bill finishes his doughnuts and rises once again from his seat.

"We'll see how they get used" he mutters under his breath. He casually makes his way to the room where the stewardess is preparing coffee. They share a sly smile. Bill closes the door behind them.

Disclaimer: None of this actually happened. I'm just poking some fun at Hillary because she voted for the war in Iraq and I'm therefore very glad she wasn't elected president.

Another Random Day At Work.

I started the workday pledged to have a new attitude. A realization snapped into my brain during the morning commute that there are kids working their ass off at college campuses across this nation hoping only to eventually have the chance to do exactly what I would be doing this day. Today, I told myself, I will honor their commitment, their hard work, and most of all their dreams. I would be a good pharmacist. I would cherish this workday.

First question: "What's the best way to remove hair from around my anus?"

Second question, asked in the thickest of French accents:

"Yes.....if I uh...kiss ze woman, who has smoked ze pot.....then I take ze, how do you say? Drug test? Do I fail?"

Yes indeed, my new attitude was paying off. Thank you pharmacy students of America, for providing me with the inspiration to get through this.

I glanced down the cleaning aisle quickly while taking a phone-in prescription and saw what appeared to be a man flossing his ass with a feather duster. It was shaping up to be an anal kinda day.

Me: "We'll have to send a fax over to your doctor's office to see if we can get you some more refills"

Customer: "But she has insurance to cover that."

Really. I didn't realize they sold those types of insurance policies, seeing as how a policy like that would be pretty pointless. Seriously, if you're paying an insurance company a premium to cover the expense of doctor refill faxes, you're totally getting ripped off.

In non-pharmacy related store highlights, a customer parked their car in front of the store's front door and laid on the horn. And laid on the horn. And laid.......on the horn. That horn got laid the way I get laid only in my dreams. An employee went outside to investigate and was presented with a demand to go back inside and get the customer some cigarettes. Reports indicated the customer was using an oxygen tank.

That's way you stay in school pharmacy students of America. Because it's better to answer questions about anal hair removal than it is to fetch an emphysema sufferers' next pack of cigarettes. I think.

As the sun set over the parking lot of my happy pill room, I took a phone call from a customer very upset that someone had stolen their medication. Friday night, stolen medication. I started to scan over the customer's profile looking for the Vicodin and/or Soma that would be too early to fill. Nope. Today was anal day:

"THE ONE THAT CAME IN THE BIG JUG! THAT'S THE ONE I NEED!!!"
"We filled that for you 8 months ago ma'am."
"I NEED IT!!!!!"

The customer was talking about a prescription for GoLytely. For those of you not in the professions, I'll tell you that the person who came up with the name "GoLytely" did it with the sole purpose of being cruel. GoLytely is indicated "for bowel cleansing prior to colonoscopy and barium enema X-ray examination." You take it the night before your examination so there's no poop in your colon any pre-cancerous lesions can hide behind, and you will not, my friends, go lightly.

Me: "Are you having another colonoscopy ma'am?"
"NO!! I NEED IT!!! IT WAS STOLEN!!!"
"Are you maybe thinking of another medication?"
"FUCK YOU!!!! I NEED IT!!!! ARE YOU GOING TO FILL IT OR NOT????"
"No, I'm not."
"ASSHOLE!!!!.........ARE YOU LAUGHING AT ME????"
"Yes. Yes I am."

And that, my friends, was the anal coup de grâce of my anal kinda day. A day that saw thousands of pharmacy students across this land doing everything in their power to someday stand in my shoes. Pharmacy students to whom I can say only one thing:

You are completely insane.

I Went Into Pharmacy So I'd Have Enough Money To Attract A Hot Chick. Oh The Painful Irony.

I'd be willing to bet that more than one of you in the profession out there may get a bit.........surly when the pharmacy goes into full scale pill moving action. You've got prescriptions coming in by phone, by fax, by electronic Rx, being dropped off in person by numbnut members of the general public. Carrier pigeons are flying in through the drive through window carrying orders for Vicodin. They all wanted their meds 20 minutes ago, and they all want to talk to you for 20 minutes.

Now I understand if you are the type of person who reads a label that says you should take your antibiotic until it's all gone and still need me to tell you in person that you should take your antibiotic until it's all gone. People like you keep me from being completely replaced with a robot. Any drug related interruption, no matter how trivial, basic, and yes..... stupid as it may be, I'm OK with. When the carrier pigeons are flying though, and you want to stop me to ask where the nearest lottery agent is, I will be mean. I have to be, otherwise nobody's drugs get out the door. Got that? It's been that way long enough now it's embedded into my very being. Non-drug related conversation = blowoff.

I found out just how deeply embedded one afternoon. I had a room full of pigeons pissed because they had to fly back to the clinic before dark. All hell was indeed breaking loose, and a woman caught my eye. Looking back I realize how hard she would have had to worked to do this. My eye is almost impossible to catch when hell is breaking loose. Eyes locked, I had to say something or look like a dork. I hoped a simple "Hi, how are you?" would let me get back to work.

"You know" she says, "I was watching you just now and you have almost perfect skin"

"Goddamn it" says the Drugnazi to himself, "I've got 30 prescriptions on the counter and an angry hoard of barbarians in the waiting room. Like I have time for this" The chick got the non-drug related blowoff, just like the lottery player.

It wasn't until the pigeons had flown off that I realized what had happened. The chick was hot. A hot chick had mounted a totally unprovoked hit on yours truly. This will never happen again, and I gave her the blowoff. This is what my job has done to me. I give the brush-off to beautiful women in order to meet the expectations of Corporate America.

I went home and drank a lot of scotch until I got sick.

The Only Other Time I Ever Came Close To Scoring At Work.

Ok this wasn't small talk anymore.......this was definitely medium talk. Holy crap this is medium talk, and I would have been more than happy just getting small talk from this woman.

I should explain. The hottest chick ever to walk into a pharmacy had just asked me where I used to work. One of the oddest things I have learned in my two decades-plus in the happy pill room is that hot women almost never get prescriptions filled. I don't know why. Maybe their hotness immediately incinerates any disease causing organisms that are deposited on their skin. Yes, there is the birth control pill, but they never want counseling on the birth control pill. Oral contraceptives are potent medications ladies. Seriously, you should talk to me about them instead of just zipping through the drive through while I am tied up talking to the woman with a beard about her foot corns.

The woman in front of me at this moment though was the total exception that proved the rule. The incredible, long, wavy, flowing red hair was just a start, I could go on all day about this woman's hotness, about her habit of showing a little more cleavage than average, about how the fact that she was indeed picking up the birth control pill took away any worries about popping out a shortie. There just wasn't very much more you could want in a customer.

She had been coming in for a few months now, and made a little small talk each time. I had learned my lesson from perfect skin woman and managed to make a little small talk back. The weather....traffic.....sports came up once I think. But I'm pretty sure her question about where I used to work qualified as medium talk. Whoo-Hoo me...things were looking up.....

"I used to work in (*insert name of poverty ridden ghetto town here*)" I reply.

"Oh, I bet you like it a lot better here away from all those disgusting Mexicans" she says in an incredibly sweet, soft tone. She honest to God thought that was a flirtworthy line.

I'm lucky I didn't implode from the change in air pressure as my hopes to score with hotness deflated at a record pace. I'll admit I briefly considered making a move anyway. I have pretended to be a Christian before in order to score, so pretending to be an official racist wouldn't be that far of a stretch. Then I remembered how the deal with the Christian lady ended, and knew that this woman's thoughts made her ugly. Crap.

She would make a hell of a stripper though. In a perfect world she'd be taking it off for pesos.

So The Hot Chick Thing Might Not Have Worked Out Yet, But Pharmacists Do Make Decent Money. Here's One Reason Why.

"Yes, I'm calling to get a refill of my blood pressure medicine." I could have just done what the woman wanted and filled her blood pressure medicine. One more prescription to get credit for and one more sale in the cash register. That's what I'm here for you know, just to put pills in a bottle.

Instead my super-spidey pharmacy sense kicked in.

"Well, I see we haven't filled these for you since October, has everything been going alright with your medicine?"

"Oh yes, it seems to work just fine, it's just that I don't need it that often"

Yes. This was definitely going to be a case for Superpharmacist.

"Hmmmmmm......well, blood pressure is usually a type of condition that's treated all the time....."

One of the reasons I make so damn much is because I know stuff like that.

"Well sometimes it gets up over 150 you know. And I'm scared I'm gonna have a stroke or something."

"I see, well do you have a blood pressure machine at home?"

I will point out again, I could have just filled her pills. That's all she was looking for. If I had just put some pills in a bottle I would have had a happy customer.

"Uh-huh. I usually measure it once a week or so, and most of the time it's OK, but sometimes it gets up to 150 or so."

"Well it's normal for a person's blood pressure to go up and down over the course of a day. The problem is when it goes up and stays up"

"Really?"

I'll also point out, that I was putting other people's pills in their bottles the entire time this conversation was going on.

"Oh sure, your doctor probably told you something like that when he wrote the prescription." I needed to find out where the hell the doctor was in this mess.

"He said he wasn't sure if I was gonna need 'em or not, but honey, he went over everything so fast, I can't remember half of what he said." So now I knew. The doctor's role here was similar to that of a sperm-chucking father, in that he started the process and then was nowhere to be found the next time he was needed. I was on my own here. So was she. That's why I now became a honey.

"I tell you what."

57

"OK...." I could hear the happy anticipation in her voice that someone in a white coat was actually going to give helpful guidance. I could have told her to hop up and down on one foot and cluck like a chicken at that point and she happily would have.

"Take your blood pressure a couple times a day here for the next few days. Mix it up.....sometimes in the morning, afternoon, sometimes in the evening, after eating, before eating, you get the idea, right?"

"Oh sure"

"Keep track of it in a notebook or something, then call me back in a few days and we'll figure out what to do about these high blood pressure pills"

She called me back a few days later and had better blood pressure readings than I do. That's why I make so goddamn much. Not because my blood pressure's higher than hers, but because I can figure out when it's best not to make a sale.

Now why mail-order pharmacists make so much I have no idea. All those fuckers do is put pills in a bottle.

Echos Come Up From The Basement Of My Brain Sometimes.

I don't know why. They just do. Miscellaneous thoughts or feelings that didn't quite gel at the time, but weren't quite forgotten. Like a Christmas present from your uncle you're not quite sure what to do with. Except it's like the Christmas presents come up from the basement where they've been stored and pop up on your kitchen table every once in awhile.

Day of Rage. That's what popped up on the kitchen table of my brain one day for no particular reason. I remember hearing something about it on the news years ago and thinking I was gonna have to look into it. The term just sounded so cool. *Day of Rage.* If I remembered correctly it had something to do with Palestinians being a little sick of the uninvited guests who showed up on their doorstep after Hitler tried to kill them all. Sure enough, I did the Google thing and discovered The Day of Rage was declared in the Holy Land on December 9th of 2000, just as I would have been settling into my new California home. Honestly I have no idea what all the fighting in the Middle East is about, as it is obvious to me California is the promised land. Yosemite, redwoods, Hollywood, sun and sand and oceans and mountains and all the food you can eat from the Central Valley. Oh, and deserts too. Just like in the Middle East if that's your thing.

I am jealous of one thing though. I want a Day of Rage. Mine wouldn't have anything to do with Middle Eastern politics though. I think my Day of Rage would be declared against health insurance companies. Me and any of you that want to join me could get us some of those cool Yasser Arafat head scarves and some slingshots, and we'd ride up to insurance company headquarters and let the stones fly, breaking many windows.

Then Aetna or Humana or somebody would come at us with a tank, and start firing rubber bullets. But we'd be like, "Fuck you Aetna. We're tired of your shit. Eat a rock bastards!"

And they would indeed eat rocks. Many rocks. And not just Aetna.

After our Day of Rage the corporate media would have to pay attention to us, at least for a little bit, if for no other reason than because Aetna and the rest of their ilk would have to explain to their shareholders why they spent money on tank deployment. We could use the opportunity to explain that $31.18 a week to make sure every old codger in this country gets the medical care they need is a bargain, and that bargain's got nothing to do with the private sector.

I didn't make that number up. $31.18 a week is what I chip into Medicare. And that covers 43,000,000 of this country's oldest and sickest citizens. If you're not a pharmacist, you're probably chipping in far less. Go look. And while you're at it compare what you're paying Medicare to how much you're paying Aetna or some other insurance company to pretend to cover your healthy ass.

After we had a chance to make our case to the corporate media, Aetna and their ilk would be shamed out of business and Medicare would be expanded to cover the entire population, saving everyone money and boosting quality of care. That's right bitch. I said saving money and improving the quality of care. Any of you right wing corpo-stooges want me to prove it you just drop me a line. I'll warn you though, you better ask politely. You come in my house with any of that Rush Limbaugh attitude and I will get out my fact claws and tear you to shreds.

Anyway, that's my Day of Rage. I might have to go down to the basement and see what else is there.

Highlights From A Random Day's Pill Counting Action

I always wanted to make some sort of mix tape of the random noises that are left on the store's voicemail overnight. That is how I start my day. Listening to the random noises. A lot of times it's the tones of someone trying to punch in a refill number. More often than I can count it's a befuddled "uuuuuhhhhhhhhh" followed by silence and a click. Once I swear it was just 15 seconds of slurping. Today it was someone singing the Hall and Oates classic "Maneater"

"Ooooohhhh-ooohhhh here she comes/watch out boy....she'll chew you up....."

Someone sang that into the store's answering machine. Listening to it is how I started my day.

I decided to test a new theory today. Whenever someone decided to interrupt me filling your prescription by asking the location of some product in the store, and I had no idea where the product was, I just sent them as far away from the pharmacy as possible, on the assumption that either; 1) They would find what they were looking for while making their way to the store's far corner, or 2) They would come across a store employee whose responsibilities actually include stocking the shelves. It seemed to work out pretty well. Only one person came back to the pharmacy to ask again, and I was on the phone and didn't have to talk to them. I couldn't believe it took me so long to think of this.

Actual conversation with a doctor's office:

Doctor's office: "Hi, I'm calling to authorize some refills for John Smith's Protonix."

Me: "OK"

Doctor's Office: "So, how many refills should we give him?"

For those of you not familiar with the process, it is traditionally the role of the doctor to issue a prescription, the doctor having been the one who's examined the patient and in theory the person with the slightest idea how serious the patient's stomach condition might be. I said 12 because it was the first number to pop into my head. I thought the lady at the doctor's office would stop and ask me why I thought 12, at which point I would sarcastically rip into her for being dumb as a doornail. She didn't. John Smith got 12 refills. Some doctor out there feels comfortable having this kind of medicine practiced in his name.

Please don't tell me you don't realize the name "John Smith" was made up. Back to the day's action:

Someone asked me where the paternity tests were while they were holding a baby. They had quite the sense of urgency. It would have made for the best video blog post ever. Moving on......

"Hi.....uuuhhhhhh....yeah.....this label says not to take if you're allergic to shellfish.......but I have high cholesterol...."

I waited for the string that would tie that sentence together. It never came. The statement was already nicely bound up in some sort of point deep inside the customer's brain. The fact that it was bound in a way utterly incomprehensible to anyone else didn't matter. He knew drugboy would make it all better.

Another customer tried to forge a prescription for Patanol. Patanol is an eye drop used to relieve allergy symptoms, and some customer thought it would be easier to try to pretend they were a doctor phoning in a prescription for it than to contact their actual doctor. Their eyes must have been itching crazy bad.

Yet another customer asked me if he could eat hot dogs if he was taking Viagra. I was able to dig out the point here. He saw the warning on the Viagra label about nitroglycerin and thought it might apply to the nitrites in his wiener.

Not his Viagra wiener. His ketchup and bun wiener. See why I had to go to college for so long now? It's important to keep the wieners straight. Which is where the Viagra comes in. OK, I gotta stop. I'm killing me.

Speaking of wieners, I can't get that Hall and Oates song out of my head now. Or maybe the term "douche bag" would apply more to Hall and Oates. I'm not sure.

I Hate Independent Drug Stores.

Why? A little story from today's pill counting action will explain why.

The Drugnazi was about half an hour behind getting people's crap out the door. The "high priority" stuff sat unmoved for longer than that, waiting for me to complete the "super high priority", "ultra high priority" and "extreme high priority" tasks that were in front of it. The phone was lit up like fucking Christmas. We were using the exact number of labor hours our corporate overlords had budgeted to take care of our customers. Just another day. Eventually I got around to answering one of the calls on the fucking Christmas phone and hear:

"Hello......this is J from Non-Corporate pharmacy in the next town over.....calling for a prescription transfer"

The voice was sweet and pleasant. It was the first time all day I had not heard hostility in a voice and it made me immediately hate her.

Our computer was on the verge of crashing and while I was waiting for it to show some sign of life I asked her how things were going. It would be better than silence I thought. I was wrong.

"Oh the funniest thing happened today. One of my regular customers sent over some flowers."

Some days, if I make it through an entire shift and never have an interaction with a customer that doesn't involve the f-word, I consider it a success.

What was slowing down my computer was the arrival of a batch of messages from corporate headquarters. They set our labor budget week by week, and next week we would have fewer hours to run the store. Another piece of me died while the friendly neighborhood pharmacist on the phone waited patiently for me to get my shit together. Bitch.

Listen up independent drugstores. I am a mean, vicious, petty man. That is why I hate you. If I have to be miserable under the yoke of corporate capitalism, then everyone has to be miserable. Got that? Damn you for being human, for treating customers as humans. You can compound your "bioidentical" bullshit estrogen to try and stay afloat all you want, but you are doomed in this era of cutting our way to every last possible dollar of profit. People must be treated like cattle, do you understand? Cattle!! One need only look to the airline industry or call your insurance company help desk to see the glorious future the free market will bring us.

Wait...

Sigh.

Any of you guys hiring?

One Day I Received The Coolest Excuse For Not Showing Up To Work Ever

"Hello, Drugnazi?"

   "Yeah, R, get your ass in here, we're getting killed"

   "I can't come in today"

   "DAMMIT!! What are you doing to me here? I thought we were friends"

   "Yeah, well, I just got out of jail."

   "Seriously?"

   "Yeah"

   "Whoa, you mind sharing here?"

   "Um, well......I was in a car with some friends, and we were driving through (*insert name of affluent lilly-white town full of old people with corks up their asses here*) and we got pulled over. It was bullshit. And the cop had an attitude....."

   "And you got into it with the cop?" I knew R had a temper.

   "yeah"

   "You fucking rock! Take the day off"

   "I'd come in, but I'm kinda tired. I didn't get much sleep when I was in there"

   "Don't worry about it. We'll get by"

   "Thanks"

So the rich old fucks who called the cops because my tech's radio was too loud ended up having to wait twice as long for their Viagra today than they would have otherwise. Justice, oh sweet justice.

   He's a good kid. Plus he's in the Air Force Reserve, which makes him a troop you have to support. Ha ha.

   It wasn't a bad day at all really.

Pharmacy In The Poor Side Of Town

I work in the affluent side of town these days, but I once spent a few years working the overnight shift in the ghetto, and I enjoy the occasional assignments that take me back to my ghetto pharmacy roots. Being a unilingual gringo, time spent in the Latino part of town can be the closest thing a retail pharmacist gets to being left alone to work in silence. Yeah, people are talking all around me, but I have no idea what is being said, allowing me a rare day of focusing on prescriptions as opposed to "WHERE ARE THE KLEENEX???"

By the way, I think "unilingual gringo" would be a really cool name for some sort of awesome sex game.

Most of this morning was spent in the noisy silence that belongs to one who does not speak the native language. About dinnertime though, a car pulled up to the drive through with what evidently was a happy sort of fellow behind the wheel.

"YADDA YADDA BLAH BLAH WORDS GRINGO DOESN'T UNDERSTAND" said the driver. This set off a sort of verbal explosion with the technician manning the window, who then said something like:

YADDAYADDAYADDABLAHBLAHBLAHYIYIYIYI
WORDSUNILINGULAGRINGOWOULDN'TUNDERSTAND
EVENTHOUGHUNILINGUALGRINGOWOULDMAKE
THEMOSTAWESOMESEXGAMEEVER
YADDAYADDAEYYIIIEYYIII
EYIIIIIIICARUMBBBBBAAAAAAAAAAA!!!!!!!

Although I'm paraphrasing here, I cannot overstate the emotion with which these mystery words were delivered. The customer then said very softly:

"yadda yadda. words gringo doesn't understand."

Then drove away.

"Um, V, is there something you want to tell me?" I said as the customer turned into the alley behind the building.

"These fuckers make me so mad!" said V, who proceeded to storm off to the bathroom.

I learned from the clerk manning the cash register the conversation went something like this:

Customer: "Yeah......I'm here to get my druuuuuugs.....some heroin.....my cocaine....."

V: "YOU STOP RIGHT THERE!!!!!! THIS IS A MEDICAL PHARMACY AND YOU WILL TREAT THIS PLACE WITH SOME RESPECT OR YOU WILL LEAVE!!!!!!"

Customer: "I'm sorry ma'am, we were just trying to be funny"

The most awesome customer takedown ever, and I missed it because I'm cursed with being unilingual.

I'm also very cunnilingual, but most, including myself, would consider this a good thing.

I really need to learn Spanish.

Pharmacy In The Rich Side Of Town.

THERE'S NO WAY I CAN JUSTIFY THAT MUCH FOR SOME MEDICINE!!!!! said the selfish milfish Mom. Then the cellphone came out. That wonder of modern life, the cellphone. It can solve any problem by getting you connected right away to a machine that will spend the next 20 minutes telling you how important your call is to it and showing you by not answering it.

It was Sunday. The doctor was out having a life. The cellphone wasn't going to solve this problem either.

ISN'T THERE SOMETHING ELSE YOU CAN GIVE HER THAT'S CHEAPER??!!?? Said the selfish milfish Mom. "Her" in this case being her daughter, who was standing right next to her. The daughter who was hearing all about how Mom couldn't justify paying for the Levaquin that would treat her sinus infection.

I should point out here that Mom's handbag probably cost as much as three or four Levaquin prescriptions. I'll also add that the last time I had a sinus infection, I would have let the doctor cut off my left testicle to get some relief, so I knew the kid was miserable. Think the girl in *Little Miss Sunshine*, except maybe 14 years old and past the point of realization that she had no business in a beauty pageant. That was this kid.

After the cellphone failed to solve anything, and after being told that matching the right antibiotic to the right bug is a matter of clinical judgment for a prescriber, which is why you have to be examined by a prescriber before you can get an antibiotic, and that no, I, who did not examine anybody, could not just pull the cheapest antibiotic off the shelf and hand it over so you can get those new shoes at Macy's, Mom left in a huff. The daughter came back alone a few minutes later with two boxes in her hand.

One contained Airborne, which is some sort of herbal mixture that at the time came perilously close in its advertising to claiming it could stop the common cold. The other was a private brand imitation Airborne. She had a check from Mom to pay for the Levaquin, but if I were to tell her that either of the Airbornes might help, she was prepared to buy one with her own money and forget the antibiotic. If it had been a little quieter in the store you could have heard my heart break for this kid. I know all about trying to win the approval of an irrational parent. I wanted to tell the kid that the good news was that eventually she'd be able to break away from the family that made her feel guilty for being sick.

As it was I told her tactfully that she was past the point where the Airborne would do any good. I didn't mention we're all past the point where

Airborne will do us any good. That point doesn't exist. All the scientific evidence would suggest that eating the cardboard box Airborne comes in is equally as effective as taking the tablets that are inside. The kid asked for a pen to make out the selfish milfish Mom's check and I reached into my lab coat and handed her one. I noticed too late it was my Viagra pen. DAMMIT! I never let the Viagra pen anywhere near a customer!! It's the only one I have left! How the hell did it get in my lab coat!!?

A little chuckle as the kid saw the logo. "You could totally sell this on eBay I bet"

"You can have it"

"Really?"

"Sure, I got plenty. Spend this much and you oughta get a free pen"

And the dorky kid with the sinus infection who I knew felt miserable smiled and said thanks.

I think I did OK that day.

Pharmacy Where The Worlds Of The Rich And Poor Intersect.

About a quarter 'till closing I hear the "rustle rustle rustle....." of a dude fighting with his backpack in the customer waiting area. The island of affluence where I sling the pills these days long ago ceded a beachhead to a homeless encampment. Usually however, they don't cross over the line into the land of the moneyed unless they're stealing booze. I figured the guy would have to have some pretty big cajones to not at least go to the back if he was swiping something, so I didn't give him a second thought. Besides, I had shit to do before closing.

Phone rang. I heard more "rustle rustle rustle...." while I advised an old woman if she could have a glass of wine with her Benadryl. I looked up and the homeless dude was at the counter. Ten till closing now. Goddamn it.

"Can you tell me how much these would be to just fill half of 'em?" He asked, and handed over three prescriptions. "I have this" and added a prescription savings card from my employer.

Missing more than a few teeth, stunk to high hell, a prescription for spironolactone and a big 'ol belly that made him look pregnant. Those of you in the professions know those last two things meant he was just about ready to finish drinking himself to death.

To which I can hear the chorus of voices saying "who cares." Fuck you. There's not a person reading this who hasn't made choices that could have turned around and bitten them in the ass at some point. This guy got bit in the ass by alcoholism. There but for the grace of God go I. And you.

A middle aged potbellied man came to pick up his daughter's acne antibiotic. Potbelly from fat, not liver ascites. He bitched about the $7 copay until past closing. That's how the twelve hour days usually end. Some fatass bitching about his copay. Today I had three more prescriptions to do.

They were cheap. Each of them right at my employer's minimum charge. I went ahead and filled the prescriptions in their entirety because I'm not supposed to go below my employer's minimum charge.

Not cheap enough for the homeless dude though. "I've only got $20 with me. I guess I'll check back with you later"

Fifteen past closing now and I got another look at that belly that looked like it was gonna pop.

"Sir did you say you just came from across the street?"

A look of confusion.

"Because we'll match prescription prices if you can find a lower one. So they just told you these were on their $4 generic list, huh?"

I was nodding my head yes.

He gave me a smile.

Lucky me had to delete the prescriptions and fill them over from the beginning. Because my employer has the most non kick-ass prescription filling software in the world. I realized what I was doing probably wouldn't put them in a position to update it anytime soon. Half an hour past closing and I got a death glare from the assistant manager who wanted to go home and a "you're very kind" from the man who had none.

I don't have to tell those of you in the profession we are the doormat of healthcare. That the fatasses bitching about their $7 copay usually come after twelve hours of other assorted cretin customers, dickhead doctors, and numbskull nurses bitching and moaning about something over which we have no control. All the responsibility, none of the control. I always said that should be the official motto of pharmacy.

I've also always said though, that every once in a while, me and the Cleveland Browns can win one. That night ended with a win. Making that night's scotch celebratory, and not an effort to wash away the day.

Two Tales Of Life For An Increasing Number Of Americans In The New Normal Of The American Economy.

So the little shit didn't seem as bad as most of the feral child-beasts that run around the store. At one point he was sitting in front of the reading glasses trying them on and checking himself out in the mirror. A four year old kid with a mullet trying on some spectacles can be kinda funny to watch actually, but man, it seemed like this little dude had been hanging around the store a long time, and, now that I thought about it, I'm pretty sure I saw him yesterday too.

Then H comes down the aisle. I'm not sure what H's job is, she changes the prices for the things that go on sale or something, not really my concern. When the little boy saw her, and yelled out "mommy!" I had my explanation. H either couldn't find or afford day care for little mullet-head, so she brought him into the store to keep an eye on him while she did her price thing. For eight hours. Putting aside the incredible boredom mullet-head must have felt having to kill all day in a drugstore, obviously giant corpo-pharmacy can't have it's employees bringing their kids to work every day to be turned loose amongst the merchandise. If whatever day-care problem H had wasn't worked out by the time the manager got back from vacation, she would probably have to start staying home. Corpo-pharmacy misses her work and she misses a day's pay. So not having a sane daycare system in place that working-class people can access makes sense how exactly?

Then there's J. She's a pharmacy tech that started a few months ago. J and I worked together a few years back at another corpo-pharmacy chain. She was an OK tech, a little annoying, but adequate enough to get the job done. When she applied to work at our store she said that she had to take some time off to take care of her dying father. Federal law requires a company to offer at least an equivalent position to an employee who takes a leave under these kind of circumstances, and they did, 20 miles away. J doesn't have a car. She does have an autistic child, and now that she had a new job, she had a 6 month waiting period to be covered under our health plan.

J had issues. Those issues, however, were being taken care of thanks to appropriate medical care. You never would have known about the issues if she had been able to afford to keep buying her meds. She thought she could make it 6 months without the medicines she couldn't buy. She was wrong. I watched her slowly deteriorate until one night she became so unhinged I sent her to the back to pretend to work on some computer training crap.

Couldn't send her home, no car. I kept going back to check on her and begged her to just let me lend her the money to buy her damn medicine for the month, but by this point she was so out of it she couldn't see anything was wrong. They let her go the next day, turned loose on society with all the demons in her head now out and raging in full force. The good news is that now that she is unemployed and unemployable, she'll be able to qualify for public assistance, which means that surely she'll soon get that car she needs. Probably a Lexus. Just ask any white-boy pharmacist son of privilege and he'll never hesitate to tell you all about the welfare people he's seen driving to his store in a Lexus. Anyway, now that J will be on welfare, feel free to hate her. I know how you upper middle class people love to feel better about yourself by hating the people on welfare.

So because of this dog-eat-dog, kick down/kiss up society that Reagan and his spawn have built for us corpo-pharmacy can't find people to do needed work and people who want to work have to stay home to take care of their children and fight the battles raging in their skulls. Thing is, these are just two little reflections of what we've become. There are other, bigger ones. You probably don't need me to tell you about a place called Iraq.

It's morning in America Reagan said.

This Looks Like A Good Place To Put In A Day's Worth Of Pill Counting Highlights.

Holy bejesus I hadn't been cut off in traffic like that in years. A full-scale, California-style I'm not gonna look cause you're gonna stop cutoff. The kind of thing I did all the time when I drove a piece of shit. This person was hellbent on getting somewhere in a hurry, and I began to fantasize about following them to find out what could possibly be so urgent. And to beat the shit out of them. My fantasy was becoming reality with every turn however, as it gradually became apparent that the piece of shit was desperate to get to......my own little happy pill room. When I saw him waiting for me to unlock the gates, I did what I normally do in these situations. I went to Starbucks and was 15 minutes late.

Turns out he was a tweaker looking for some Sudafed. God I miss the days when heroin reigned supreme. Heroin addicts are much better drivers, even if they do tend to be a bit slow.

The label printer started the day printing everything about a half an inch below where it should be. Supertech tried valiantly to fix things, but seeing as we were already 20 prescriptions behind, we didn't have the luxury of being able to do a full-scale printer takedown. I suggested we call our corpo-pharmacy technical support desk and we both had a good laugh.

People from the corporate mothership were here to help though. Some dude in a suit was leading the store manager around making her write things down on a clipboard. They got to some little shelf-thingy next to the pharmacy register and suitman wasn't happy at all. "Drugnazi, didn't we get the end piece for this display in our last order?" nervously asked the store manager. "I'm pretty sure we did."

"I don't know" I replied. "I don't pay attention to that stupid thing" and I think I heard suitman audibly gasp. I learned later he was some sort of Vice-President. Evidently in charge of little shelves.

The label printer was now printing everything half an inch above where it should be. "Can't you just go back and undo half of what you did?" I asked Supertech. Her look told me to back off now.

The next customer at the counter handed me a piece of paper on which a Nurse Practitioner had written these words exclusively ...."Needs malaria pills" I assumed the Nurse Practitioner was stupid enough to think "malaria pills" were over the counter. I was wrong. The Nurse Practitioner charged the patient $30 to write out a note the Nurse Practitioner intended the patient to give to her doctor. Who would then probably charge the patient another $75 to write out another note the patient would then give to me so I could sell her some Malarone and be reimbursed by her insurance company for $2 more than the Malarone cost me.

At least the customer wasn't on welfare though, Because getting the shaft business-wise from Medicaid is way worse than getting the shaft from a private insurance company for some reason. Plus then I would have had to notice what kind of car she was driving. It's some sort of requirement that drug store employees take careful notes on the type of car everyone on public assistance drives at all times. I'm glad Malarone lady had Blue Cross, as I was too busy to follow her out to the parking lot.

Michael Bolton came on the store radio, and I knew it was a sign my label printer would soon be working good as new. Even though I had just heard Supertech cuss for the first time ever.

"Take one capsule at bedtime" read the next prescription. USE SPARINGLY was in caps and underlined. It was made out for 45 capsules with 5 refills.

Later on, I filled a prescription for a child whose actual first name was "Rum".....and the printer alignment gap narrowed to about a quarter of an inch. Supertech was defeated. She dialed the number, incorrectly it turned out, for tech support on the speaker phone......

"LIVE.....HOT......LOCAL.....LADIES!!!!!!" blared out of the speaker phone for those in the waiting room to hear. I made a note of the incorrect number.

I also came across a way cool disease name. Sick Sinus Syndrome. I think it would be cool to go around telling my friends that I had Sick Sinus Syndrome. Or maybe name my band "The Sick Sinus Syndrome"

Half an hour before closing time the labels started to print correctly. The next to last customer at the counter asked me how much they should feed their new cat. I was able to answer her. The last asked if I had to go to college. That's the absolute best way to be my friend. Ask me if I had to go to college. I said no just to fuck with him.

If I remember correctly the shelf thingy got fixed way before the printer. Release the Scotch.

The End Of The Drugnazi

The Doughnut hole. No, I'm not talking about that thing you put around your bat when you're on deck in baseball. Neither am I talking about bite-size goodies you load up on when you're at the Krispy Kreme. Those of you in the profession know exactly what I'm talking about. For those of you who aren't, I'll let you know the "doughnut hole" is a term that refers to a coverage gap in the Medicare Part D drug plan. In a nutshell, Part D covers you for awhile, then stops, then starts again. It's stupid, but that's not the point of this post.

The lady at the counter was in the doughnut hole. She came in the store to get some medicine to treat a brain tumor. For just shy of a thousand dollars, chances are she would get to live about an extra 2 months.

Label popped out and I saw the price. Then I looked over and saw her sitting patiently by the blood pressure machine. Fuck. I hate this part of the job. I waved the cashier away because I knew I should break the news myself. It's almost a relief when they yell at you in these situations. It's when they're just quiet and hand over a pile of cash that you feel like shit.

I took a deep breath and started. "Mrs. Smith, I don't know if you knew this, but this medicine is pretty expensive........."

She heard me out and didn't bat an eyelash. Then she took my hand and said something like "The last 60 years have been a gift young man" At least I think the word she used would translate as something like "young man".

Then she gave my hand a pat, turned her arm over, and I saw the blue numbers tattooed in her skin. This woman had been a concentration camp inmate. I looked up and our eyes locked for what couldn't have been more than a few seconds. It felt like an hour. When I saw those eyes I saw a wisdom, a confidence, and an inner peace that I do not have the ability to put into words. This woman was tougher than any drug bill. She handed over a pile of cash and I felt like shit.

As she left I wanted to run after her and ask her to tell me something, anything, about what she had been through so that maybe I could help keep some part of her story alive. I didn't. I stood there like a moron as she walked out of sight and I haven't seen her since. Months after she left all the sudden I couldn't stop thinking about her. It's funny how a memory can go underground and then pop right back up with the right trigger. So, um, yeah, even though it was a retreat from my battle against growing up, I decided I didn't want to be the Drugnazi anymore. Not that I felt all that different about most of humanity mind you, I just thought maybe there could be a better name out there. I like monkeys, so I thought something monkey based. Maybe The Drugmonkey. I decided to try it out to and see if it stuck

A New Name Changes Nothing About My Typical Workday.

I had been in the happy pill room not 5 minutes when someone asked for my opinion. About the new Diet Coke with lime. I figured what the hell, the credibility of five years of college coupled with passing a licensure exam ought to count for something, so I gave him my opinion. I've never had lime flavored Diet Coke in my life, but I told the man it was good stuff. People like it when you keep things positive.

Later on an actual real medical doctor did ask for an actual real medical opinion. My answer was interrupted by a man shouting at the top of his lungs that he needed a carburetor for his car.

It's important to point out here that he specifically said it was for his car, as they started using fuel injectors in place of carburetors in automobiles around the time Reagan became president. It's also worth noting that they were never sold in drugstores. I'm really glad they did away with the glass enclosed pharmacy. Otherwise I would miss out on the carburetor questions and have to listen to the doctors instead.

I am so done with perfect skin woman. She came in that day and she had cut her hair. What once was long and flowing to the middle of her back did not now even reach her shoulders. I'm going to grow a big zit in retaliation.

Actual question from an actual customer: "Is tetracycline bad for you?" Someday I will answer such a query with a simple "yes"

I had an actual customer with an actual first name of "Memory." She was dropping off a prescription for Aricept. The prescription was for her mother, but it was still pretty funny. Aricept is for Alzheimer's disease.

The lady with the Percocet prescription was in soooooooooooo much pain she had to wait right by the cash register so she could have it as soon as possible. She literally moaned when Supertech told her it would be 20 minutes to fill the prescription and begged us to do it sooner because she was in so much pain. Then she parked herself right in front of that cash resister and waited through thick and thin. Through screaming babies and angry fellow customers who didn't appreciate her being 12 inches away. Through phone calls and insurance rebills, through a 10 minute discussion with a man about the best type of water pik to use, faithfully she waited by the cash register.

Until the cashier told her the Percocet was ready. At which point she decided to run to the other side of the store to get some Doritos. I can relate, although the kind of hurt for which I find Doritos to be effective is usually emotional.

More Evidence Your Prescriptions Cost So Much Only Because Of The Massive Amount Of Research Dollars That Went Into Developing The Product.

So awhile back I was doing my online travels, which naturally lead me to the website of Allergan Inc. Allergan is the leader in eye care medicine, and I am nothing if not a fan of eye medicines and stuff.

Or maybe I was doing research on my secret project involving botulism toxin. I'll never admit which one it was.

Allergan, you see, is the manufacturer of Botox, a form of one of the most deadly poisons known to the human race. It has some medical use in the treatment of problematic eyelid spasms, and it can also be injected into the skin of a cougar (an old horny woman, not the member of the cat family) to give her a better shot at landing a young piece of beefcake by making her skin look less wrinkly. There were rumors John Kerry used it during the 2004 presidential campaign as well.

Anyway, guess which form of Botox Allergan cares far more about? Hint. Did you even know it had a legitimate medical use before I just told you?

"So typical of Big Pharma" The cynical Drugmonkey thought to himself as the Allergan webpage loaded. I knew the score though. A Pharmaceutical Corporation's goal, like that of any corporation, is the accumulation of as many dollars as possible.

But then I saw this, the opening paragraph of Allergan's homepage:

> Allergan, Inc. is a multi-specialty health care company focused on discovering, developing and commercializing innovative pharmaceuticals, biologics and medical devices that enable people to live life to its greatest potential — to see more clearly, move more freely, express themselves more fully.

Gasp! Allergan had changed! Their focus, the very first thing they say, is enabling people to see more clearly! Move more freely! Express Themselves! A president who isn't dumb and a Pharmaceutical company committed to enabling people to live life to its greatest potential all in the same year! My God! It truly was a new world!

That paragraph was located right next to an ad for Allergan's new product, Latisse, and I wondered if perhaps this Latisse was a miracle cure for Trachoma. After all, eliminating the world's leading cause of infectious blindness would definitely help people see more clearly, anyone who isn't blind could most assuredly move more freely without one of those guide dogs, and not having to wave around a red-tipped cane in front of you would probably let you express yourself better. A perfect fit for Allergan's stated goals! Plus, a better plan to treat Trachoma, which has blinded 8 million people worldwide, than the current one, which is basically blanketing a town with the antibiotic azithromycin once an epidemic has taken hold, would give Allergan bragging rights over those cocky bastards over at Pfizer. A win-win for everyone!

Of course you can also stop Trachoma, which has infected 84 million people, by building a town a basic sewer system. But that's effective and cheap and doesn't lead to resistant strains of bacteria you can make more money off of later by inventing new antibiotics. Plus it makes people think about poop, and who wants to think about poop? Anyway, I was convinced this Latisse would just have to be something like a new, vastly improved treatment for Trachoma as I clicked on the ad to find out all the details:

You couldn't click on the ad. I had to use Mr. Google, which led me to the answer. Latisse was the first FDA approved medicine to treat.....

...thin eyelashes. I shit you not. Millions of people blind in this world because they don't have a place to poop and Allergan is very proud of themselves for finding a way to make their eyelashes thicker. Which when you think about it, might actually work against Allergan's stated goal of helping people see more clearly depending on how long and lush those lashes got. Drat. Big Pharma lied to me again. At least we still have a president who isn't dumb.

"Drugmonkey, you corporate hating commie, you're not being fair!" I can hear some of you saying. Latisse is another version of Lumigan, the glaucoma medicine, Allergan does have a commitment to help people see clearly!

And your facts would be correct. Latesse is the exact same thing as Lumigan, which costs around $80 for a 2.5ml bottle. Allergan plans on charging $120 for a 3 ml bottle of Lumigan with a different label. So yeah, I guess while they do have some sort of a commitment to helping some people who are rich or insured see clearly, they also have a commitment to ripping you off. Which is what I call charging 37% more per milliliter for the same stuff.

There's no commitment whatsoever to the African villager looking for a decent place to shit however. No commitment from anyone. He'll take his dump the best he can and be blind someday. Enjoy your Big Pharma $120 a month body-altering mascara women of America, and remember always the reason prescriptions cost so much here:

All that cutting edge research that keeps getting done.

Yet Another Random Workday

The heat slipped into the pharmacy this day exactly the way mustard gas would choose to. Slowly. Seeping through the vulnerabilities of the building's insulation systems steadily and without mercy. Wearing away our comfort like the drip of Chinese water torture, which I forgot there for a second was renamed Chinese enhanced interrogation method by the Bush administration. Once a year, twice at most, it gets hot enough in my city that you might want air conditioning. Which means once a year, twice at most, we are reminded that my employer's air conditioning does not work. So once a year, twice at most, a member of management calls an air conditioning repair company who shows up and makes loud banging noises on the roof for a few hours. By the time the banging noises are made however, days have usually passed, and it has cooled down naturally, meaning there is no way to test that the banging noises were effective. Around a year later, my employer finds out the previous summer's banging noises accomplished nothing. Today was such a day.

The printer broke too. Which means I had, on average, to print 5 labels for every one that I could use.

The first words out of the mouth of the first caller of the day: "I DON'T KNOW WHHHHAAAAAATS GOING ON HERE!!!!!!!," and I could not have agreed more. I was immediately convinced, before the second sentence ever came out, that the caller, indeed, had no idea what was going on. In any aspect of their life.

He was out of refills and didn't understand what the words "no refills" on the label meant. The fact he looked at the label at all put him in the upper 80th percentile of my customer pool.

We had fans in the pharmacy while the rest of the store's employees did not. Because we are not stupid and they are. I took comfort in this and in the fact that warmer weather meant the chicks were wearing less clothing. I swear I saw areola at one point. I thanked the nipple Gods.

A prescription was presented for fluconazole 125mg, use vaginally at bedtime. Fluconazole is an oral tablet that is not made in a 125 milligram strength. I broke the news to the customer.

YOU HAVE NO IDEA WHAT IT'S LIKE TO HAVE VAGINAL ITCHING!!!!!! It was yelled. At the top of her lungs. And while I had to concede that the customer was correct on that point, I also had to explain that volume would not make her doctor clarify this turd of a prescription any faster, especially when directed at someone who did not write the prescription and who had no prescribing authority. I did much better with the next person to yell something out.

MY BLOOD PRESSURE IS 47 OVER 20!!!!!!! I NEED TO GO TO THE ER!!!!!! I sprang into action. Even though I am not qualified to practice medicine, I went through an objective diagnostic procedure. It went something like this:

I see sir, that you are an idiot.

Using the store's blood pressure machine takes, although a limited amount, some brainpower.

If your blood pressure were, in fact, 47 over 20, you would be dead. Or at the very least unable to yell at me while I am on the phone with a doctor.

Conclusion? You fucked up taking the reading. Savings to the health care system? Probably a thousand bucks or so if the person were on Medicare. Seventeen hundred if he was covered by a for-profit insurance company, who would have then immediately terminated his coverage.

You're welcome America.

Unfortunately it was now time for lunch, and to face my fear.

The lady at the fast-food Chinese restaurant has been giving me things. Last week she didn't charge me for my meal. A few days later she brought me over a newspaper and didn't want it back. Yesterday she threw in a bowl of soup. I don't understand, and quite frankly, am afraid she at some point might expect repayment in non-monetary ways, which wouldn't be so bad if she were attractive. At all. This whole situation has been a source of great amusement to my staff. After areola woman left I asked, "Why can't a woman like THAT ever give me soup?"

"Hahahahahahahaaaaaaaaaaaaa"......said my technician. "No soup for you." She is unaware of Seinfeld, and how she made the Drugnazi thing come full circle.

She was also right. I chickened out and went to Subway. As the sun relented from providing the days heat, I thought of the annual banging of the air conditioning ducts and of the orange chicken I would never have again.

Why Do I Hate Fake Boobs?

I'll tell you why I hate fake boobs. Because there is a woman somewhere out there who put her hope in a bottle of iron tablets. That's why I hate fake boobs.

I suppose I should back up a bit, lest you think the Drugmonkey has spent another lonely night with his friend Mr. Scotch. It all starts when a woman comes up to the counter and asks what kind of vitamin might be good to take to help a person's energy. Every pharmacist has been asked this. Here's how the conversation usually goes:

Me: Most of the time a person feels run down it's because they're just working too hard, not getting enough sleep, stressed out, that kind of thing, and there's not really a vitamin that's going to help with that. There are times when a vitamin deficiency can make a person feel tired, but it's usually a case of a person pushing themselves too hard.

About half the people will stop here, agree that they are indeed working too hard and stressed out, and leave with a smile on their face. People take acknowledgement that they are being run into the ground as one of the most wonderful complements they can receive.

The other half goes into "I am going to buy something no matter what you tell me" mode. Every pharmacist is familiar with this as well. Getting some rest is anti-American on so many levels. Not only are you not working hard when you give your body time to recharge, you are not buying anything, thereby contributing to the downfall of western civilization just as surely as Osama Bin Laden himself. These patriotic Americans get the "it's possible a deficiency in iron or vitamin B could cause a person to be chronically tired, however, YOU SHOULD HEAR FROM A DOCTOR that this is the problem in your case before you try taking anything." speech

The customer, having been instructed on a possible way to spend money, will never fail at this point to immediately go to the vitamin aisle, and the lady tonight was no exception. She returns shortly with a bottle of iron tablets and one more question:

"There's been a lot of blood when I poo-poo. Will these help with that too?"

Ok, this is serious now. This woman needs a DOCTOR, and the Drugmonkey tells her this in no uncertain terms.

She gets very quiet, then asks, "Do you know where I could buy health insurance?" She was probably undocumented, and obviously a pretty recent arrival, but knew enough about the system to know uninsured = screwed.

I tell her about the low income clinic down the street, the one that hasn't been able to keep its doors open on a regular basis since the regular doctor left. I think he burned out. I don't really blame him. She gave me a quiet thank you and I knew that she was going to take those goddamn iron tablets hoping they were going to fix everything.

As she walked out the door, I thought of this guy I knew in college. Maybe the only person I've ever met whom I might say is as smart as me, he went on to med school, and, as some of you might have guessed already, is now a plastic surgeon. Last I heard he limited his practice almost exclusively to rich women whose self esteem can be tied to having either salt water or a silicone/oxygen polymer placed under their boob skin. "That way I don't have to deal with the riff raff" he told me the last time I saw him.

It's a lot easier to hold the riff raff in contempt when you don't have to look them in the eye. I couldn't get that woman's face out of my mind for days. I may be the only one who cared about her and I couldn't help.

I hate fake boobs.

This Is Getting Depressing Again. I'll Lighten Things Up By Turning A Chapter Over To My Store's Laser Printer.

First off, let me just say I understand the pressure a modern pharmacy is under. To compete in today's prescription drug market one has to be ruthlessly efficient, focused as much as possible on meeting the needs of the customer and providing them with a satisfying health-care experience, while at the same time eliminating non-productive activity and redundancy.

I know you don't believe this right now, but I am here to help.

Do you realize I can print prescription labels almost 10 times as fast as the dot-matrix model with which you had the good sense to replace with me? And not only that, my labels are crystal clear, and far easier on the eye, giving your establishment an aura of added professionalism. There is, no doubt, a reason why those old models can be had these days for less than the cost of dinner at the local burger house.

Excuse me, but there seems to be something jammed just above my duplex. Would you mind opening me up and clearing that out? I'm afraid I will be unable to work until you do. Thank you very much.

Now, where was I? Oh yes. I'm sure you'll agree the additional speed and clarity.....

Oh dear, I'm sorry, but evidently there was an additional paper jam behind the toner cartridge. How embarrassing. If you could just open me back up we'll be back at work in no time.

ALT ERROR 846: unknown transfer origin.

How odd. Neither me nor anyone at my manufacturer's help desk seem to have any idea what that could mean. Perhaps you could look in my owner's manual if I came with one. How about we just hit the "clear" button and pretend that never happened.

Now then. As you are well aware I'm sure, I also have the capability of doing far more than printing prescription labels. I also quickly and efficiently print a drug monograph for every prescription you fill, putting vital information into the hands of your customers and enabling the FDA to require a never ending expansion of the number of medguides to be supplied to your customers. I hear one may be coming soon to warn of the risks of the allergy medicine Clarinex, which is slightly more dangerous than water.

I understand your frustration sir, but just as soon as you replace my toner cartridge with a new one, my work will look as good as the day I was installed, making that type of language completely unnecessary. Be sure to box up the old cartridge and send it back though. They are expensive, and I would hate to see you lose your rather substantial recycling deposit.

I haven't even mentioned my ability to print out e-prescriptions and faxes, creating a giant pile of different sized papers you have the opportunity to sort through while quickly trying to put each customer's prescription information in the proper bag. I honestly don't know how you got by back in the day when items from different sources and of different priorities actually printed in separate, pre-sorted places.

ALT ERROR 846: unknown transfer origin.

I told you earlier sir; I do not know what that means. Perhaps it has something to do with the persistent black streak I have been putting down the center of the last 200 pages.

ALT ERROR 846: unknown transfer origin.

ALT ERROR 846: unknown transfer origin.

ALT ERROR 846: unknown transfer origin.

I understand you have a dozen customers waiting sir, but there really was no need to slam the paper tray back in me so hard. Let's think about all the time and money I save you the 80% of the time I am working.

Pardon me, do you smell something burning?

EXCUSE ME! Now kicking my sides is completely uncalled for! I'm afraid if you do not bring your temper under control I will have no choice but to repeatedly overload the circuit breaker that services your entire computer system. Trust me sir, neither one of us would want that.

Because that would stand in the way of progress.

Thank you for understanding.

One More Random Christmas Memory.

The holidays.....oh if we could only keep that Christmas spirit flowing all year long. Celebrating the Big J's Birthday by pretending, if only for one month out of the year, that we give a shit about the message he was trying to send us. January through November we may adhere to the dog-eat-dog creed, but for that one glorious month we all rejoice in the fraternal bonds of our shared humanity.

Like this customer who came to the counter one day as the season drew near. He was full of the Christmas spirit. He was truly excited about his favorite time of year, and asked me about my holiday plans.

"I'll be right here" I said. Which was the truth. Corpo-Pharmacy was dumb enough to offer double time for filling 10 prescriptions and I was dumb enough to cash their check.

"Oh that's terrible" he said, very concerned for his fellow human being. "It's not right to make people work on Christmas"

"I don't mind" was my reply. "I'll just buy myself something nice with the holiday pay" Which again was the truth. Visions of scotch were dancing through my pharmacy brain.

There was a slight pause in the conversation. "What are you, Jewish?" the lover of humanity finally replied. His voice suddenly dripped with absolute contempt.

Now I have a sister who's into the genealogy for whatever reason. She's traced my DNA back to the whitest country on earth. I went to a Presbyterian church when I was a kid and it was while attending a Methodist college that I became an atheist. So naturally I answered the man's question with the words;

"Yes. Yes I am"

"Figures" He says. Then he turns away and mutters something about Hanukkah. I never saw him again. I seriously think he never came back in the store because he didn't want to do business with the dirty Jew boy.

The day before this happened I would have told you there was nothing left the general public can do that would surprise me. I suppose it's a testament to my glow in the dark whiteness that that day I was proven wrong.

I wonder how hard it would be to burn a Star of David on someone's lawn.

The Anti-Semitism Will Make A Nice Segue Into Another Workday Story.

"No Arabs will come to this store again!! We will not do business with them ever!"

Believe it or not that customer statement cleared up a lot of confusion on my part. I couldn't for the life of me understand why this man cared so much where his cephalexin came from, but the second he heard it was made by a company called Teva, he hit the roof. This kind of thing usually only happens with the narcotic seekers, who are very specific as to the manufacturer of the pills they want, as they want the same letters and numbers to be stamped on the tablets each time they have a prescription filled so they can assure the people they are selling them to that they are not ripping them off.

But Teva, as some of you in the profession might know, is headquartered in Israel. A country that can ignite passions stronger than even an opiate addiction. This is why I don't have cable my friends. I was witnessing a combination of CNN and Comedy Central right in front of my eyes for free.

Except the cephalexin was prescribed to treat his daughter's ear infection. Which made the episode a little tragic as well.

So anyway, according to Abdul the Arabs are done with my store. Somehow we'll just have to get by. I hear the Jews have all the money anyway.

From knowing too much for your own good to not knowing nearly enough. Feeling generous, I asked the nice old lady customer if she would like me to ring up the other items in the cart behind her along with her prescriptions.

"I don't know" the nice old lady customer said. "Is that my cart?" She seriously had no idea. Cart determination took a good 5 minutes. That was the reward for my generosity. Lesson learned.

About an hour later a man came up to the counter with the cotton part of a Q-Tip stuck in his ear. Deep into his ear. Evidently I was the only Emergency Room in his PPO network or something.

The next person told me they needed a 20 inch Ace bandage and asked if the one labeled "Fits 18 to 21 inches" would work. One extreme to the other seemed to be the theme of the day.

Around midday a customer told me there was once a NASCAR driver named Dick Trickle. I didn't believe him, but I thought it kinda funny anyway. As the usual assortment of prior auths, refill too soons, and why is my copay so highs piled up, as I spent my day with three people simultaneously demanding my immediate attention while my own dick yearned to trickle, every once in awhile, I would think of a race car driver named Dick Trickle and chuckle. I went home and looked him up. Dick Trickle is real, and after the morale boosts he gave me that day, I cannot help but to believe he is a force for good in this world.

Of course the day ended with a customer dropping off a prescription at around the 11 hour and 59 minute mark. "The nurse at the emergency room said I should come here because the wait at the other store is always so long." Such was my reward for not being a fuckup.

I thought of Dick Trickle, and ended my shift on a note of happiness as I dispensed the last of the day's Jewish antibiotics.

After Today, Whatever I Accomplish In My Life, For Good Or Ill, Will Be Because Of One Man And One Man Only

The day started with Supertech calling in sick. Supertechs by definition don't call in sick until they are ready to die, but I had no time for sympathy. The replacement cashier sent by the overlords of retail to replace 20 years of pharmacy experience started the shift with these words:

"How do you run this cash register? It's different from the ones up front."

I hoped Supertech wasn't too sick, mainly because the last thing I needed was for her to come in here and add another goddamn prescription to my misery. It was a pill blizzard of the worst sort my friends. I triaged and triaged and triaged again and if you had a kid screaming because he felt like someone was driving an icepick through his eardrum and inching it into his brain you were still looking at about an hour's wait. Partly because I was simultaneously performing the duties of pharmacist and corporate cash-register trainer. Partly because of calls like this one:

"IS THIS THE PHARMACIST???" The customer had specifically asked to talk to the pharmacist. He had waited probably a good 5 minutes for the chance.

"Yes it is, may I help you?"

"DO YOU HAVE A DRIVE THROUGH?"

I should make clear here that the customer did previously talk to a human that they decided wasn't qualified to handle this question.

"No we don't sir""

"THE PHONE BOOK SAYS YOU HAVE A DRIVE THROUGH"

"Well I can't speak for what's in the phone book, but I'm here now, and I can tell you there is no drive through in this building"

"HOW AM I SUPPOSED TO GET MY PRESCRIPTION FILLED?"

He went back on hold. I remembered that night after I got home that I never talked to him again. I wondered if he was still waiting for me to pick up the line.

He might have been the man who came in about an hour later and said he was lost. Not that he didn't know what part of town he was in, but that he couldn't figure out how to get out of the store. It was obviously starting to frustrate him. I told my wonder-boy cashier to stop staring at the check he couldn't get the cash register to accept and get the old coot out the door. He later reported to me the man asked if he could walk him to his car. Which he then drove away.

I was pulled from the sea of prescriptions again for this question:
"How often do I take this? I don't like reading all these labels and stuff"
That wasn't even close to the stupidest question of the day.

After about 7 hours of this, of me and the cashier boy and 5 phone lines, a fax machine, and a constant angry lynch mob breathing down my neck, I could feel a wheel start to wobble on the finely tuned pharmacy machine that is me. I'm no stranger to hot lynch mob breath in that sensitive spot under your ear, but this was different. There are times when I can actually feel blood pouring out from my wrists, and I assume that's not a good thing. Mr. Drugmonkey was getting ready to crack.

Then I heard it.

> *And I'm proud to be an American,*
> *where at least I know I'm free.*
> *And I won't forget the men who died,*
> *who gave that right to me.*
>
> *And I gladly stand up,*
> *next to you and defend her still today.*
> *' Cause there ain't no doubt I love this land,*
> *God bless the USA!*

The absolute worst part of the worst song ever recorded wafted over the store's radio system, through the chaos of the pill room, and into my head. I hate how he says he won't forget the men who died and the implication that any women killed in the service of the American Empire he loves so much aren't worth the effort it would take to remember them.

And I really hate that song. For so many reasons. I could write a whole other book about why I hate that song.

So you know what I did? I bucked it up. You wanna know why? Because when I finally snap, I will at least have the pride of knowing that it wasn't some no talent, sap-sucking, tone deaf, twit hacking up simple-minded jingoistic bullshit for the Reader's Digest crowd that pushed me over the edge. When I lose it, there's gonna be a quality soundtrack in the background.

I decided that if a soulful jazz number came over the store's radio system, I could finally let go. It never did, and all the prescriptions eventually got out the door.

Lee Greenwood saved my life.

Another Reason Your Prescription Costs So Damn Much. My Interview With The Antibiotic Doryx.

Me: Thanks for making the time to come in today Doryx, I know you're a busy drug.

Doryx: Thank you for having me Drugmonkey, and for the opportunity to explain why my unique enteric-coated pellets of doxycycline hyclate means there is no substitute for me!

DM: Meaning if your doctor writes a prescription for Doryx, it cannot be filled with any other type of doxycycline.

DOR: That's right!!

DM: What did people do before you came to market?

DOR: Well they didn't get the benefit of my unique enteric-coated pellets, that's for sure!

DM: No, seriously, what did they do?

DOR: Got by with outdated versions of doxycycline the best they could I suppose.

DM: And did these old fashioned versions of doxycycline have some sort of problem with bacterial resistance, or another sort of effectiveness problem that necessitated your invention?

DOR: My niche is more on the safety side Drugmonkey, you see, my enteric coating means I don't start to dissolve until I pass though the low pH environment of the stomach and into your intestine, and if I don't start to dissolve until I pass through your stomach, the chances of me triggering stomach cancer and leading you to a slow agonizing death would seem to be almost nil. Did you know stomach cancer has one of the lowest survival rates of any malignancy?

DM: Are you saying other forms of doxycycline cause stomach cancer?

DOR: Well I'm not in a position to comment on what other doxycyclines might or might not do. All I'm saying is that I never touch your stomach. I also contain no uranium, which means the chances of me becoming fissionable material and triggering a thermonuclear reaction are pretty much zero.

DM: So Doryx could be an integral part of a nuclear-free world?

DOR: Absolutely.

DM: I see. So while we're on the subject of safety, do you cause less fetal harm if given to a pregnant woman than regular doxycycline?

DOR: No.

DM: Less photosensitivity?

DOR: No.

DM: Less Clostridium difficile associated diarrhea?

DOR: No.

DM: Less....

DOR: Look, I'm enteric coated, OK? I think the benefits of that would be self-evident.

DM: So self-evident that it's not really necessary to do any actual scientific studies to quantify what these benefits might be?

DOR: There are limited research dollars for these type of things you know. I think we can all agree that our resources are best spent elsewhere.

DM: Speaking of limited dollars, you are aware that a month of Doryx therapy can cost over $500?

DOR: I'm glad you brought that up Drugmonkey, the people at Warner Chilcott, who make me, are very concerned about the impact of high drug prices on patient care. That's why we've developed a Doryx Savings Card program. Once enrolled in this program, a patient will pay no more than $25 dollars for a Doryx prescription, cutting the retail price by over 90%!! Those are real savings for real people.

DM: For the first three months.

DOR: Well, yes.

DM: And with how you've positioned yourself as an acne medication, as opposed to an antibiotic to treat acute infections, you expect most of your customers to take you for far more than 3 months, don't you?

DOR: Unless they want their zits to come back and end all their chances of ever being accepted by the cool kids in school.

DM: And you know a month of regular doxycycline costs less than $15.

DOR: Look, I know our time is running short here, but ask yourself, if your tumor-laden stomach were to explode in a toxic mushroom cloud, how much would you have paid to prevent that? There are some things you just can't put a price on Drugmonkey. Thanks again for having me on.

DM: We.....um...actually have plenty of time left.

Doryx bolts out of the studio......

———

Disclaimer: There is no link between any form of doxycycline and stomach cancer. That was just a fictional example of the kind of bullshit I imagine Doryx would say if it could talk.

Another Random Day Of Pill Counting Highlights

It was 9:30 and I was worried. I had taken the usual opening flurry of phone calls, which were, in order, people checking to see if their Vicodin, Valium, Soma, Vicodin and Vicodin were ready to pick up, but none of them were from John. I checked the calendar to make sure it was Friday. Never had I worked at this store on a Friday morning and had John fail to call to check on his Vicodin by now. I briefly considered the possibility that John had finally learned that not once had any of these calls resulted in anything other than "it's a little too soon to fill that John"

Briefly considered the possibility I said. I knew it was more likely that something had happened to John. I hoped he was OK. He really isn't that bad of a guy.

The Friday controlled substance extravaganza continued as the next person at the counter had their prescription denied by their insurance company. It was Friday, so I assumed it was a refill too soon. You know what they say about assume. This one was a "drug not covered"

"But.....but.......what do poor people with no insurance do?" said the customer with the newly acquired interest in his fellow human beings.

"Not get prescriptions for Ambien, that's what they do, because they have to save their money for when they're really sick and not for when they just can't fall asleep" was on its way from my brain to my mouth when a recall was issued. I decided if a sleepless weekend was what it took for this man to become aware of the insurance crisis in this country, then me being a smartass probably wouldn't help anything. I listened to him as if he were Lou Gehrig telling Yankee stadium he was the luckiest man on earth.

Lady with poison oak: Do you have any recommendations?

Me: Put some hydrocortisone cream on it.

Lady with poison oak: Is there any kind of cream I could put on it?

Sometimes the only reason I don't kill myself dear customer, is because that would mean you won.

A call came in around midafternoon. Thank God, John was all right. He's an electrician you see, and his work took him out of town this week. Another drugstore was calling for a transfer of his Vicodin. I told them the last date of fill assuming it would sink in.

Me: I don't think you'll want to fill that one.

Them: There are no refills?

Me: There are, but he got a 30 day supply a week ago.

Them: What?

Me: It's too soon to fill. You don't want this one. This guy's got a history.

Them: Can I have your DEA number?

Me: Hang on.

Then I put the other drugstore on hold and called John's cellphone. It was way easier to explain to John his prescription was too soon to fill than it was this dumbass at the other drugstore. John understood right away. I left the other drugstore on hold until they hung up.

Half an hour later I accidentally called someone the name of a famous porn star. Whoops. It was close to the customer's actual name though.

Last prescription of the day was a woman who couldn't remember her child's date of birth. She knew it was the 30th. No doubt in her mind on that one. She kept going back and forth as to whether it was January 30th or April 30th though, and she couldn't remember the year for the life of her.

"She's 18 months old" was the best she could do. Maybe I really wouldn't be the world's worst parent.

Oh, and I saved someone from a phenobarbital overdose. They totally would have died if the prescription would have been filled as written. The fact that that felt like the most insignificant part of the day was the main reason it was washed away in a river of scotch.

More Evidence It's That Expensive Research That Drives Drug Prices.

I looked at the advertisement that had been designed just for people in my profession. It showed three bar graphs, the last of which was much taller and a bright orange, as opposed to the plain black and white of the other two. That bar represented Glumetza, and it was obvious this new med was way better than its competition. I mean seriously, all you had to do was look at the graph. You'd have to be stupid not to realize how much better Glumetza was.

Glumetza, however, is simply an extended-release version of the diabetes medicine metformin. Remember the ER trick I told you about earlier? Here was a prime example. You can probably find metformin on some drugstore's four dollar generic list, while a month's worth of Glumetza will set you back around sixty. This was a little different though, as the message in this ad was that Glumetza was actually more effective, not just more convenient. All you had to do was look at the graph. The Glumetza bar was taller and the numbers at the top are way bigger. And orange as opposed to black and white. That's all you needed to know. No need to read the fine print, where it clearly said they used a daily dose 33% higher to get that pretty full color bar.

No need to think about how maybe it's not all that surprising that when you give a dose of a drug that is higher, it might be more effective.

Here are some other tidbits from the text of that same Glumetza ad:

> Unlike generic immediate-release metformins, Glumetza uses advanced polymer technology, which provides controlled release of metformin targeting the upper GI system. As a result, more drug enters the bloodstream and less unabsorbed drug remains in the lower GI tract. This may help reduce GI adverse events.

I see. Well I think Glumetza may make your penis fall off. And I have provided as much proof for this claim as Santaris Inc. and Depomed, the makers of Glumetza, did for theirs.

In the clinical trial above, Glumetza was well tolerated
at higher doses. The overall incidence of drug related
AEs (adverse effects) was 35% for Glucophage (*the
brand name for regular metformin*) 1500mg/day BID
(*twice a day*) and 33% for Glumetza dosed up to
2000mg QD. (*once a day*)

Sweet. A 2% reduction of the chance of any side effects is totally worth
paying $660 extra dollars a year for.

The numbers above regular metformin's bar on the graph just weren't as
big though.

Less than 1% Glumetza patients discontinued
treatment due to GI AEs in the first week of the study,
when the assigned dose was 1000mg/day.

Except that big bar on the graph was for a dose of 2000mg/day. Santaris
Inc. and Depomed didn't seem to want to mention how many people
discontinued treatment at this dose. So I'll just assume it's somewhere
around 95%.

Sigh. You know, the fact that a drug manufacturer massages some
numbers around isn't what bothered me. Drug manufacturers have
massaged numbers around at least since I was a drunken frat boy. They used
to be far sneakier about it though. Now it's like they don't even care, and I
miss being respected enough that they would at least try to spray some Lysol
on their bullshit. These days it's like Big Pharma is giving bulls a special diet
to make their shit extra stinky or something.

And evidently the extra stinky bullshit works on someone out there.
Because I filled a prescription for Glumetza later on that day. That's what
bothers me.

An Open Letter To My Cat.

You've been here a few years now, and you may have noticed that there are parts of our home that are carpeted and parts that are not. Do you think that next time you cough up a hairball, that maybe....just maybe..... you might just consider leaving it somewhere on the 50% of the place that has bare floor? Just once? It might make for a nice change.

And what's with the way you chew my stuff? Holes in my clothes, bedsheets, furniture, even your own freakin' bed. I thought that kind of shit was for dogs. I was very clear at the SPCA that I wasn't interested in a dog, so seriously, there's no need for any inferiority type complex.

I also shower every day, making you licking my arm in the middle of the night when I'm trying to sleep completely unnecessary.

On the other hand, meeting me at the door when I come home from a day of dealing with pill-seeking barbarians is kinda cool. Feel free to continue this.

And the way you fall asleep on your back with your paw raised in what looks like a black-power salute is pretty funny, although I doubt you're aware of the political statement you're making. Oh hell...........never mind you furry freak. Just please stop chewing on the electrical cords. You might end up killing us both.

Perhaps I Should Have Gone The Extra Year For My PharmD. Degree.

I have a five-year Bachelor of Science in Pharmacy degree you see. I had the option of going to school an extra year to earn a Doctor of Pharmacy, or PharmD, but couldn't see the point of another year out of my life and another year of tuition payments for zero extra qualifications to enter the drugstore life.

The day came though, when I questioned the wisdom of that choice.

It wasn't the first question the customer had that stumped me. He said he was going to Yosemite and wanted to know what he should get in case he came across some poison oak. Wake me up out of the coma-like sleep you will likely find me in most days around noontime and I would be able to answer this one before fully waking; "Hydrocortisone cream and Claritin" So far so good.

It was the next question that stumped me. The customer now wanted to know about bears. Namely, what he could buy to prevent a bear attack. I seriously think he was convinced a bear might be waiting for him at the park's entrance station. I went over the options in my mind:

Tylenol- May be useful *after* an encounter with a bear. Like maybe if the bear knocked you down while he was running away from something else.

Benadryl- Not so much.

Milk of Magnesia- Not quick acting enough to distract a bear intent on mauling you for your picnic basket.

I briefly considered Neosporin, like maybe filling a bathtub full of it, before realizing that again, this would only come into play post bear attack.

I looked up and saw a giant display for the new diet wonder drug Alli, but it would also be of little use. Alli is known for a side effect euphemistically known as "anal leakage," and I don't think you'd need much help shitting your pants if you were face to face with a bear.

In the end I advised the customer, who I should add was doing his camping at the Yosemite Lodge, that the best course of action would be to take basic precautions to minimize the likelihood of a bear encounter, like not keeping any trash in your car, and sticking to places bears are likely to avoid, like the area around Yosemite Lodge, which when I was there had the feel of midtown Manhattan with a waterfall in the backyard.

The customer and I both ended the conversation with the feeling we had just talked to one of the stupidest people on earth.

I really should have gone for the PharmD.

A Guest Appearance From Yohimbine, The First Prescription Impotence Medication.

I never meant for it to go so far. I am so sorry.

When they came to me and asked me to play the role of a chemical that could stimulate a man's penis, I'll admit, I thought it was a big joke. I was young and stupid and just didn't realize there was a demand for that sort of thing. I knew I didn't work, but I assumed everyone else would know that too. And then there was the FDA. Weren't they supposed to keep ineffective drugs like me off the market? Surely they would step in and keep things from getting out of hand. This all must be some sort of prank I said to myself. I'll just have some fun while it lasts.

I'm not sure when exactly I saw the first wrinkly old man face looking to me for hope. I'm sure I didn't notice it. The money started rolling in quick and it all seems like a blur now. The parties at oceanside mansions, the powdered blow in the bathroom, the oral blow in the bedroom. The butler and the maids. The separate Rolls-Royce for each day of the week. I don't remember a lot about the 70's, but at some point the wrinkly old man faces became too numerous to ignore.

"Yohimbine you can save my marriage." They would say. "Yohimbine, you can make me a man again. Please help me"

I tried to wash away their pleas with vodka. With gin, rum, scotch....anything.....anything to make it go away. Two stints in The Betty Ford center didn't help, because the problem was I was living a lie. I wanted out. All the money in the world couldn't buy back my soul, but there were contracts. Obligations to which I had committed myself. The day they started running that ad in pharmacy journals with the little male symbol, the circle with the arrow... the way they made the arrow gradually start to point upwards. That day I wanted to die.

The wrinkly old man faces never stopped. No matter how many times I failed them, they always came back with more dollars in their hand and more hope in their hearts. They were looking to me to restore their masculinity, but if I had been any kind of a man myself I would have put a stop to it.

It was a relief the day Viagra came to market. When the vultures and hangers on and groupies finally abandoned me. Things are better now. I live in rural Pennsylvania eking out a living as a seldom used pupil dilator. Every once in awhile I still run into someone who believes the myth, but now I can tell them. I won't make your dick hard. Neither will I burn fat if you apply me to your skin as a patch. I won't. I never did.

I'll never be able to undo the damage I did to the wrinkly old men. The only thing I can do is ask their forgiveness, try to be the best pupil dilator I can be, and hope that you can learn from my mistakes.

Please, if someone claims you can cause an erection, demand scientific proof before you sign any contracts.

Sincerely,

Yohimbine

Viagra Chimes In.

Yo, Yohimbine,

I saw your letter while looking around the Internet for sites that try to make a buck off my good name, and I gotta tell ya, I feel for you man. You're one of the few chemicals on earth who can understand what it's like to be me. It's hard. Actually in your case it wasn't hard, but don't beat yourself up about it, OK? Without being able to see and learn from what you went through back in the day who knows if I could handle being me.

The fame.

The never ending geyser of cash. Never ending I said.

The women. And not just women mind you, if you swing that way, there's the men, transsexuals that could be either one even. Fuck dolls. Pocket pussies, watermelons, oak trees, plaster of paris sculptures, electronic devices, certain types of desserts and egg products. It never stops. If I hadn't married Ambien a few years back I might never get any rest. She's been really good for me, that Ambien wife of mine.

Anyway, my point is we all stand on the shoulders of giants, and you did some good pioneering work. I owe a lot of my success to you my friend.

Even though we work in totally different ways. As a matter of fact, our mechanism of action isn't even close. Now that I think about it, you really had nothing to do with the research that created me. I owe way more to people looking for a way to combat chest pain. I started off as a heart drug you know. I was about as effective at preventing angina as you were in making a stiffie, but those heart researchers never let me give up. Yeah. A drug like Imdur is probably the giant upon whose shoulders I stand.

Never mind.

Sincerely,
Viagra

While We're Talking About Penises, A Plumber Made Mine Shrink One Time

2 weeks ago- The filth came out of my tub like the primal oooze of a swamp in Louisiana. I've only been to New Orleans, and never to a swamp, but I'm sure this is what a swamp would smell like. The ooze isn't the problem though, it's normal when I haven't run the bathtub tap in the second bathroom for awhile, and being a shower man, the only time I run it is when I think I might have a guest over.

Notice I didn't necessarily say overnight guest. It's best not to probe too deeply into what goes through my head sometimes:

"Well hi Bob, it's good to see you stranger! How you been? Would you like a cup of coffee or a bath or something?"

The ooze wouldn't leave though. That was the problem. It set up camp at the base of my drain and refused to budge.

Naturally, the first step was to jiggle the drain lever thingy. It was jiggled. The ooze let out a mocking, sinister, laugh. I saw some screws and took them off. My tool set consists of some Philips screwdrivers, a pair of needle nose vice grips I found in a parking lot once, WD-40, and some packing tape. Not even duct tape. Packing tape. That tells you how seriously I take my tools. This ooze situation reminded me of many a Saturday afternoon around the house with my dad fetching tools. At my place I can say "Could you get me the vice grips?" When I was a boy around the house though it would have had to have been far more specific. Something like "Hey boy, while you're sitting there resting, get me the blunt nose single sply quarter turn 45 degree upward angle alloyed vice grips"

When I returned it would be something like "The single sply! You think I can take off this engine block with double sply vice grips? The biggest part of a project is having the right tools boy." I was referred to as "boy" or "the boy" until I was around 15 I think.

So I matched up the situation to my tools and took out some screws. Then I looked around. I sighed impatiently at the ooze to let it know it was now time to leave. When I stared banging on whatever was a couple inches below the drain I knew it was time to stop. My brother in law has a plumbing business, and I'm pretty sure I heard him say once at Christmas that everyone's presents that year were financed by husbands who started banging on stuff. I used the last tool in my tool box and a tactic a friend of mine uses when he has house guests. I put a roll of toilet paper within view of the ooze.

"I'm glad to see you. I said to my guest. But when it's gone so are you"

1 week ago- The fatal flaw in my plan has become evident. Plumbing ooze does not defecate and therefore has no need for toilet paper. So now it evidently thinks it has an invitation to stay until the roll naturally decomposes over the course of the next few hundred years or so. I can't help but to think if only my vice grips were single sply the problem would be solved. As it is I come to grips with my need for professional help and can feel my penis shrink a bit as I call the plumber. The lady who answers the plumber's phone is very nice and has a sweet voice, exactly how I imagine the receptionist would sound at an impotence clinic. I swear she's ready to say "It happens to every guy eventually" as she leafs through the appointment book.

"I have a spot open for 8 AM" I wait for the list of later times I'm sure is to follow. None do. The thought I could easily live with just one bathroom floats through my mind. I take the 8 AM appointment confident the plumber will arrive late.

Yesterday- I receive a request to get a picture of the plumber's crack while he's over.

Today, 8:01 AM- The phone wakes me from a dream in which my mother has just been chosen to be a contestant on a reality TV show. I think the show had something to do with cooking. I was hoping they would have her make lasagna, as I hadn't had mom's lasagna for years.

"This is Heather from Bob's plumbing!!!" were the words that snapped me out of my pasta fantasy. "They're on their way over!!" Her name wasn't really Heather but she totally sounded like one. Heathers have a distinctive sound and I suspected it was her middle name. I decided on a breakfast of black coffee.

8:03- Plumbers arrive before any caffeine is drinkable. The main plumber seems much too skinny to have a crack. The second is very soft spoken and seems like some sort of gentle giant. If I am to get a picture of a plumber's crack this day, he will have to be the one to supply it.

8:05- Plumbers are finished. "It was either gonna come easy or it was gonna break" The main plumber told me as I struggled with the coffee filter. I imagined how it went down. "We can do this the easy way, or the hard way" he said to the ooze, then he showed it his plumbing license. The gentle giant then sat down next to the ooze and told it a story about his childhood that made the ooze realize this had all been just a ploy for attention. The gentle giant and the ooze shared a hug and the ooze went to the sewage treatment plant to face its fate like a man.

In reality the plumber said "I just loosened it up with a pair of vice grips. It's mostly about having the right tools."

I handed over a check and felt my penis shrink some more. I guess I'll take a bath now and think of the lie I'll tell my tech tomorrow when she asks how my day off was.

Why The Health Care Reform Effort Was So Important. And Why It Didn't Go Nearly Far Enough.

If the great healthcare debate of 2008 had a poster child, it would be Eric De La Cruz. Eric didn't get to dress up in a revolutionary war costume or wave around a "Don't Tread On Me" flag like the mostly healthy, mostly insured people that showed up at town hall meetings all across the country in an effort to protect us all from the tyranny of health care security that year. Making an effort to ensure our lives would never be placed in the hands of an uncaring bureaucracy. That no American citizen would face a death panel. Making sure that never happened was what the great debate that introduced most of us to Tea Party was all about. Eric wasn't into the theatrics of these meetings though. He never shouted down a member of Congress or waved around signs of President Obama with a Hitler mustache. As far as I know, he never even went to any of those town halls. He was too busy fighting for his life.   He was normal enough kid with a normal enough life, except that he ended up 27 years old and with severe dilated cardiomyopathy. Bad news the dilated cardiomyopathy is. Those of you in the professions already know this means his heart would get progressively weaker until it was either transplant or death. Eric was sick, and he was ready to do everything he could to get better. Had he been born in Toronto, or London, or Paris, or Tokyo, that would be the end of this story and I could move on to how I plan to regain my manhood after my encounter with the plumbers. Eric had the bad taste to be born in the United States though, where no private insurance company was gonna touch a kid with major heart troubles with a ten foot pole. Eric was placed on Nevada Medicaid.

"Oh, well that sounds like the end of the story then" You might be saying. "Tell us about your plan to regain your manhood now."

Nope. Because Eric was also rude enough to reside in Nevada, where there are no heart transplant centers. Nevada Medicaid will not pay for out of state care. So Eric would just have to die. Two times a court of law told Eric he was just gonna have to die. I'm not kidding.

Good thing those Tea Partiers are ever vigilant against the appearance of any death panels.

That's what happens in the hodge-podge blend of senseless private for profit and 50 separate state government run except for the parts that aren't government run programs that we call a health care system in this country. If you're in the wrong place with the wrong problem you just have to die, even if you could have lived on the other side of a state line.

Which is why I say burn it down. The whole fucking thing. What passes for a health care "system" in this country needs.....to be.....destroyed. Because what would save Eric....his only hope....was the one part of our system that is national socialized medicine. Medicare.

If Eric could get covered through Medicare, the federally run health care plan that offers universal coverage for the nation's oldest and sickest citizens for far less overhead than private plans, he could get back to only worrying about if a compatible heart would become available and the monumental task that is recovering from having a major organ ripped out of your body and replaced. Fortunately for Eric, Medicare is overseen by politicians and not CEO's. Politicians need votes, and when Eric's sister raised a ruckus about the screwing her brother was getting, the politicians realized letting one of their constituents die so publicly might not be the best way to get those votes they need. Eric was granted Medicare coverage. So thanks to his sister and the national socialized medicine part of our health care system, he had a chance.

It shouldn't have been necessary. The ruckus raising. You shouldn't have to have a sister like Eric's to have a chance to live. Because not everyone has a sister like Eric's, who was a journalist at CNN and managed to form a "Twitter Army" of supporters to raise awareness, and money, for his cause. The band Nine Inch Nails got involved, and while I've never thought of their lead singer Trent Reznor as a warm and fuzzy kind of guy, I'm glad he did.

I'm infuriated he had to though. You shouldn't have to have connections to a rock star in order to have a chance to live. I don't care who you are, if you're lying in a hospital bed and your heart is struggling to keep you alive, and if there is a therapy that has a good chance of keeping you in this world, what kind of sick barbarians would stand in the way? What kind of society would look a 27 year old kid in the eye and tell him the rules of the bureaucracy mandate that he'll just have to die?

Ours. We told him that twice. God bless America.

So burn it down. The whole fucking system. You, and me, and Eric, and everyone else in this country deserve a hell of a lot better.

Or I should say, Eric deserved a whole lot better. The sister that was a TV journalist and the rock star did manage to finally get Eric into a hospital, but he never made it out. By the time he got there he wasn't healthy enough to have transplant surgery. Eric died in July of 2009. Many people you have never heard of have no doubt died preventable deaths since.

And will continue to do so. Because after all the Tea Partying. After all the meetings and shouting and gnashing of teeth and scare tactics and politicking and bill passing and a grand signing ceremony in the Rose Garden. The same thing would probably happen to Eric today. He would still end up on Nevada Medicaid with the only heart transplant centers on the other side of a state line. After all the effort that went into reforming our "system." Nothing would have changed for Eric. Or for anyone in Eric's situation who doesn't have a media-savvy relative.

Burn it down.

Highlights From A Random Weekend Of Pill Counting.

Friday started as a day of hope. Because as you have no doubt picked up on by this point, I am nothing if not a creature of hope. Perhaps as I slept, I thought to myself, a cure for everything had been developed, rendering me obsolete in the new state of health care nirvana the world now found itself in. True, I would be unemployed, but thanks to the cure for everything I could be assured that I would always have my health, plus I could sleep in. I decided I would take that deal, and I crossed my fingers. A guy's gotta have hope.

Then I realized that even after the cure for everything was developed, my employer would still need someone at the back of the store to tell people where the bathroom was. I got out of bed and left for work.

Fifteen minutes into the workday Supertech informed me there were no bags. In the pharmacy or in the backroom. This happens a lot. The fact we will need bags to put the purchases of each and every customer that buys something into seems to come as a complete surprise to the store's management each week. Perhaps they were expecting no customers for the next 7 days. That would explain their staffing level. I walked to the front of the store, where the only non-pharmacy employee on duty was manning the cash register. I stole his bags. Right in front of him. I took them all and did not apologize. On my way back to happy the pill room I lifted the bags skyward as if they were the head of a vanquished enemy. Later on I wondered what the store did to meet their entirely predictable bag needs. I never asked, and the store's management has learned not to bother me with trivial details like the fact I steal their supplies.

As I entered the cure center, a customer was having a lengthy discussion with Supertech about whether you could tell if he was a woman dressed up as a man. "There are places in San Francisco where you totally can't tell!" he made the point with great emphasis, and while I don't doubt this is true, I couldn't help but wonder why he seemed so anxious to talk about it. On a Friday morning. This is usually the subject matter for a Friday night.

Then the same customer didn't want to touch the store's pen to sign his credit card slip because "it's diseased," leading me to believe he was still up late from the night before. His type usually aren't early birds.

Later that day I waited on a mall security guard who requested easy open lids for his prescriptions. That made me feel more secure.

Customer approaches with two bottles of Mylanta. "Which is stronger, Ultimate strength or Maximum strength?" I really couldn't blame the customer on this one. Turns out Ultimate trumps Maximum. Unless you have gas.

Sometime Saturday a man approached the counter, again with two products, one an ointment and the other a cream, and asked, "One of these is creamy, right?"

"Yes, the other would be more like Vaseline" I said.

"Well which one's creamy?"

Sometimes my friends, you will find yourself in situations dealing with the general public where you really don't want to be a smartass, but you have no choice. I didn't know how else to say it.

"The one that says cream"

"OK, thanks a lot!" said the happy customer. Like I had just enlightened him on the principle of quantum mechanics. I went to college 5 years for that. I skipped a lot of class, but believe it or not, it never catches up with me most days.

Also on Saturday a lady whose insurance claim rejected asked "Do you think it could have something to do with how I haven't paid my premium this month?" I said maybe. Didn't want to put any words in the insurance company's mouth.

Maybe that actually happened on Sunday. Hell, I can't remember anymore.

Also on Saturday and/or maybe Sunday the fat lady who waddled up to the counter said she just couldn't understand why no pharmacist she had ever talked to recommended the Hydoxycut to lose weight. Seriously, she was well north of 300 pounds. I had just weighed myself that day and discovered I'd dipped under 170. It made for such a great visual. Maybe I can steal the stores security camera footage the way I steal their bags and put in a picture if this book makes it to a second printing.

It was definitely Sunday when I had my frustrating conversation with the insurance company help desk wage slave who sounded like he was talking to me from Mumbai. Way too friendly to be an American this dude was. After mad investigation of an incredibly perplexing problem, Mr. Mumbai and I determined its source to be my employer's software. Meaning I would have to call my employer's computer help desk. My employer's computer help desk would be about as helpful at solving problems on a Sunday afternoon as my cat Spooky. "Ah shoot, I was afraid you were gonna say that" I semi-sighed. "Wish me luck."

"Very good luck on your quest Sir" said Mr Mumbai, and the weekend ended as it began, with a glimmer of hope. Not from me, but from halfway around the world. It certainly wasn't the cure for everything, but I decided I would take it.

Because I am nothing if not a creature of hope.

I Feel As If I Haven't Been Doing My Part In The Hunt For Osama Bin Laden

I mean, there's a storage unit right next door to my condo, and I haven't checked it one time since the attacks of 9/11. I have also failed to look in the wooded area between my condo complex and the highway.

I'm almost afraid to go look now because it would be really embarrassing if he were there.

"Drugmonkey, you idiot, Osama Bin Laden is holed up in the tribal areas of Pakistan, and is nowhere near your little rathole condo" some of you may be saying. To which I would reply; "If you know so much about where Osama Bin Laden is, why haven't YOU found him?" It's been almost 10 years now, so obviously it's time for a little outside the box thinking here.

Back to my point though. I'm afraid this whole Osama Bin Laden fiasco may be as much my fault as the CIA's. I'm going to go check out that storage unit as soon as I sober up. I don't think one should risk an encounter with Osama Bin Laden when even the slightest bit intoxicated.

I Live The Fantasy of Every 12 Year Old Horny Beavis-Boy. Kind Of.

I NEED TO KNOW WHAT TO PUT ON THIS RASH!!!!!!!! Said the nice lady customer at the counter. The lady customer knew that it would be very important for me to see the rash in question. The rash was under her boob, and she was absolutely convinced I had to see it.

Yes, she whipped it out. Right in front of me, my trusty technician, the store manager, and the guy who wanted to know which aisle the laxatives were on. You can imagine the attractiveness of a woman who would do something like this. You wouldn't be wrong.

Now, I could have lost it, and when I was straight out of pharmacy school I more than likely would have. Time has taught me though, that the quickest way to get that thing out of my face was to remain calm. "I don't need to see it ma'am" I said, then asked a couple questions, suggested some Lotrimin cream, and for once was happy I had a job that ensured that I had not had a chance to eat anything for the last 10 hours. She had more trouble getting it back in than she had getting it out.

Over two decades behind the pharmacy counter and now I am not the least bit fazed when a random ugly woman unexpectedly whips out a yeast infected boob. I'm really not sure what that says about where I am in life.

A couple weeks later a kid peed in front of me. He's standing there at the counter and just lets it go. He didn't whip out his wiener mind you, just went right in his pants. And it's not like he just couldn't hold it anymore and a little bit leaked out, it was Niagara Falls roaring down his pant leg........and onto the floor........and down a good ways into the first aid aisle. He was probably like 5 or 6 years old. Definitely old enough that he should have had the proper training.

His mom was there right beside him. Her reaction, delivered in a tranquilizer induced monotone: "Um, you should have told me you had to go."

Thing is, I wasn't really all that surprised. This is what working in retail has done to me. I am not fazed by seeing a little boy piss down his own leg.The boy didn't really care either. That's what the ghetto had done to him.

A Random Tribute To Whoo Guy

If you ever saw the movie *Walk The Line*, you'll remember the scene of Johnny Cash's concert inside Folsom prison. You may or may not know that that concert actually took place, was recorded live and is available from your favorite music retailer. It was one of my favorite albums back when the hipster doofuses that worship him today wouldn't have given Johnny Cash the time of day if they met him on the street. If you don't have a copy you should go buy one right now. When you do, you'll hear after Cash sings on the first track that he "shot a man in Reno just to watch him die" one of the audience members (inmates) lets out a very distinctive, and very loud, WHHHHHHHHHOOOOOOOOOOOOOOOOOOO!!!!!! The line affected this man on a very deep, personal, level, and it shows.

I often wonder what happened to whoo guy. I'd like to think that after his release from Folsom, he formed a country and western band and spent many happy years touring off the beaten path waystations with a unique musical art that while it never made him rich, satisfied his creative soul and inspired others to express themselves using their artistic gifts.

More than likely though whoo guy took a shank in some vital organ and died. He was definitely happy during his whoo moment though, and I guess that's what the concert was all about.

Sometimes The Customer Is Not The Idiot.

So I'm dragging my sorry ass into the happy little pill room one morning and hating life just a little more than usual. I'm not really awake yet. No surprise there. Some dumbfuck is waiting at the gate thinking if he stands 2 inches away in the moments before I show up to unlock it, that means his Vicodin will be done all the faster. No surprise there. What I'm dreading is throwing open that gate and seeing the mess the agency guy left for me. Agency guys suck. In an era of pharmacist shortage, when I once landed a job by sending in a postcard and showing up for an interview wearing jeans, when I got unsolicited job offers via telephone and US mail a couple times a week, agency guys were unable to land steady employment. You can just imagine then, how competent they must have been and the joy of having an agency guy at your store. And they are almost always guys. I've yet to see an agency woman. Wait. I should clarify that. I mean an agency woman who works for a pharmacy temporary placement service. Woe is the pharmacist that has the shift after that of an agency guy.

That day did not disappoint. Before I could even get to the gate I see the following note taped across the pharmacy alarm keypad:

"COULDN'T GET THE ALARM TO WORK, SO I DIDN'T SET IT. ANY PROBLEMS GIVE ME A CALL!"

I should mention that the store and the pharmacy are open different sets of hours, and that this keypad is outside the pharmacy, meaning that for 2 hours, members of the general public were walking by a helpful sign letting them know that there was no alarm guarding the room 'o drugs.

How the hell do these people get out of college?

For a couple minutes I thought about taking him up on his offer to call if there were any problems:

"Hello, dipshit? This is the Drugmonkey. Just letting you know all the Vicodin is gone. The real problem though, is that you neglected to post a sign saying exactly how much money was in the safe and the combination. Also, next time maybe you could make a banner with my home address and the hours I will be working and not at home. Not to be all negative though. The way you somehow left 20 prescriptions on the counter when we went out of our way to schedule an extra cashier for you was simply unparalleled in the annals of laziness. Should you ever be assigned to work at this store again, please kill yourself instead."

Sometimes I need a day off more than oxygen.

Sometimes The Customer Is Not The Idiot, Part Two

"Ms. Smith, it says on your new customer form that you're allergic to Lortab. Is that correct?"

"Yes"

"So what exactly did the Lortab do to you when you took it?"

Ho hum. I do this a couple times a day. I got ready to hear all about how it made her tummy hurt. Snore. The doctor who wrote the prescription for Vicodin had probably heard all this already. Sigh.

Lortab and Vicodin, you see, are two different brands of the same product. Like Motrin and Advil are both ibuprofen.

"Well, it made me really itchy, and I got these splotches...."

Holy crap! A real allergy that made its way to my level! This is like a blue moon. It happens just often enough to remind you that it can.

Stupid customer obviously didn't bother to let her doctor know.....because there's no way a doctor would write a prescription for Vicodin if she had told him this. Because Vicodin and Lortab are the same thing.

"Well, this prescription is for a different brand of Lortab....."

"WHAT!!!!????? YOU HAVE GOT TO BE KIDDING ME!!"

Turns out she had let her doctor know. And she had asked her nurse once she started itching in the hospital if they were giving her Lortab. More than once she had asked if they were giving her Lortab. Because Lortab made her itch. The way she was itching now.

Wow she was mad. Can't blame her really.

Sometimes The Customer Is Not The Idiot, Part Three.

I have long said that in every pharmacy there is one person that holds the whole place together. I have also always said that that person is never a pharmacist. Those of you in the profession know exactly what I mean when I speak of the "keystone tech." They're the ones you scan the schedule for every week hoping to see them working the same shifts as you. They're the ones who can put fear into your very soul with the mere mention that they might use a sick day, although they never seem to. The ones that know that Blue Cross of Buttfuckistan is actually billed to Buttfuck Prescription Advantage, and that you have to use "ERW&^!!!+WAGSUX #@!" for the group number, but only on Tuesdays. Every pharmacy has a keystone tech, and they are worth their weight in gold.

Unfortunately the keystone tech always seems to be balanced out by the "other" tech. Perhaps it's pharmacy yin and yang. Or maybe it's some sort of corporate tax thing, but those of you in the profession know exactly what I mean by the "other tech" as well.

Customer: Can I use your phone?

"Other" tech: What's your last name?

The type of tech who when checking in your warehouse order will take your antibiotic ear solution and make a space for it next to the over the counter earwax removal products. The fact that space had to be made in no way deterring her in her steadfast belief that nothing used in the ear could possibly require a prescription.

Someone shoplifted one of the antibiotic solutions before I realized what she had done. She's worked here almost a year now.

It's funny stuff until I lose my license. Then I will have to kill her, which is a shame because she's really a nice person.

I hope the shoplifter at least had an ear infection.

Dear 16 Year Old Kid I Never Had The Second I Got My License The Way The Rest Of My Breeder College Friends Did.

Just take the goddamn car you little shit. It's only a matter of time before you get yourself into a mess your old man won't be able to get your sorry ass out of. We might as well get it over with. Just take the goddamn car.

Do you really think I don't know what you're up to with that little ho of yours? Or that weed is odorless? Just because I'm too fucking tired to see straight after getting my head pounded in for 12 hours at the store doesn't mean I'm blind. Here's a tip; lambskin condoms don't stop AIDS. Not that I have any illusions you'll start listening to me now.

You know what I'm gonna do tonight while you're busy finding a way to wrap the car around a tree? I'm gonna catch up on all the sleep I lost walking you around in circles when you were crying with the colic. I'm gonna doze off in between sheets that aren't the least bit stained with spit up. Spit up is the most disgusting substance known to humankind, and I have seen the last of it. I'll probably be so goddamn nice and cozy I'll sleep right through the call from the sheriff's department asking me to bail you out of the pen. Think of your night in jail as the karma go round for you registering as a Republican to try and get under my skin. Christ, I wish I would have turned around and shot you on the wall. Totally, totally, wish I had never had you.

Wait. I didn't have you. I forgot there for a second. I feel better now.

Pfizer Says They Are Inspired By A Single Goal, Your Health, Which Somehow Led Then To Try To Shove Cardura Down Your Throat. Or, Another Reason Your Prescription Costs So Damn Much.

Because heart failure evidently fits in with that single goal. Your Health.

I mean, Pfizer wouldn't lie. At one time that was the first thing you saw on their web page.

"At Pfizer, we're inspired by a single goal: your health."

Keep their inspiration in mind while I tell you a story.

Many people believe that in healthcare, new automatically equals better. Even many in the professions work off that assumption. Thing is, in reality, as far as drugs are concerned, new just means better than a placebo. That's the standard a new drug has to meet in order to be let on the market. If Old Maid Drug is 90% more effective than a placebo, and Young Sexy Drug is 30% better, the FDA will more likely than not approve Young, Sexy, Inferior Drug. Guess which one Big Pharma will be promoting though?

And in most cases we would never even know that Old Hag Drug is better than Young Sexy Drug. Because the incentive for Big Pharma is to stop its studies the very second YSD is shown to be *any* better than a sugar pill, and start buying new low-cut dresses for its sales staff in anticipation of YSD's immediate approval.

Bottom Line: we usually don't have nearly enough information to know just how effective a new drug is, or how it measures up against what's already on the market. We only know that it's better than nothing.

Someone in the bowels of the scientific bureaucracy in the federal government, namely, The National Heart, Lung and Blood Institute, once had an idea to change that, or at least change a little part of that. The feds organized a huge clinical trial to rate and compare various treatments for hypertension, how effective they were at preventing heart attacks, strokes, and other cardiovascular problems, you know, the whole point of putting someone on a hypertension medicine in the first place. Everything from old-school diuretics to medium-school calcium channel blockers to new school ACE inhibitors were gonna get a look at. Even alpha blockers.

"Alpha blockers, WTF?" Some of you young whipper snappers in the professions might be saying. "Who takes alpha blockers for high blood pressure?" Well this old man's here to tell you there was a time when people did. A biggie back in the day was Pfizer's Cardura. Nice name. Makes it sound like it's gonna make your heart all durable and stuff. I bet someone was really proud of themselves for thinking up that name.

Thing is, Cardura was only added to the study after Pfizer doubled their contribution to the study's costs, from $20 million to $40 million.

"We're so inspired by our single goal, your health, that we didn't think twice about kicking in an extra $20 million to promote our single goal, your health" A Pfizer spokesman never said.

Except that when the study's data started to roll in, it showed that people taking Cardura were more than twice as likely to end up in the hospital with heart failure as those taking a diuretic. The data was so bad that the Cardura part of the trial was stopped.

Now everyone out there who thinks that this disastrous clinical data immediately led Pfizer, who says they are inspired by a single goal, your health, to stop promoting Cardura for hypertension raise your hand.

Ok, everyone with your hand up, I've been hammering away at this book for over a hundred pages now. Have I taught you nothing?

What Pfizer did to promote their single goal, your health, was to send out a memo with instructions on how to assure doctors Cardura was still safe.

Remember, this was after data started rolling in that was showing Cardura might not be safe.

Pfizer sales reps also kept some doctors from hearing a presentation of the study's data at a cardiology conference by arranging for them to go sightseeing.

Asked for comment, a Pfizer spokesman didn't say, "Ummmmmmmmmmm.......well......have you heard about Viagra? It makes your Willie hard and stiff!!"

Sales of Cardura held up through 2000, when it lost its patent and became an old hag, making it no longer profitable for Pfizer to send doctors to go do things like get drunk in the French Quarter so they wouldn't see actual science at scientific conferences.

Not an old hag like chlorthalidone though, the oldest of the old school hags in the trial, which was also the most effective med in preventing heart attacks, strokes, and heart failure combined. Good luck getting someone besides me to tell you that though. Use of meds like chlorthalidone rose a paltry 5% after the study.

Maybe I should get me a low-cut dress or two.

My Cat Seeks Medical Attention.

The hairballs had been unbearable, but now her mind was at ease.

The dashingly good looking veterinarian had told her that the malady was easily treated as he handed over the signed slip of paper. "Just take this to your local drugstore and you'll be as good as new by the morning." he said. Spooky had noticed a stunningly beautiful Persian cat in a business suit and a low cut blouse walking out of the vet's office as she made her way to the appointment that morning. Little did she know that was a sign of trouble. Right now though, as she made her way into the pharmacy, she felt reassured. That everything would soon be better and the constant tummy torment would soon end. She assumed the sign above the front door stood for "Cats are Very Special"

The first thing she noticed was a line at least 20 deep waiting to get to the drop off window. It made her want to take a nap. She woke up 2 hours later and the line was now down to 15. Eventually she made her way to the counter and was told it would take at least an hour to fill her prescription. She started to softly purr.....

"Is there any way you could get it done sooner? Look how fluffy and attractive I am. Surely a creature so cute should not be made to wait more than 10 minutes"

She was then told it would be an hour and a half.

She let out a hiss, and was then distracted by an open plastic bag being blown down the antacid aisle. Must chase the bag.

The bag was captured and hidden inside of for a good 10 minutes, which left 80 more to kill. On her way to the other side of the store to shoplift some catnip she stopped twice for emergency grooming.

She talked to no one this whole time. My cat is a total bitch. Once she got high off the catnip she sat on her paws with her back to the rest of the store.

Not that she wasn't pleased. The fact that it was stolen made the catnip high all the better, but eventually her tummy was rumbly again and it was the time the prescription was promised to be ready.

She waited 2 more hours to get to the pickup window. It was then she learned a trick to use when dealing with the Cats are Very Special pharmacy. If you immediately walk over to the pickup line as soon as you are done dropping off your prescription, by the time it is your turn it will be past the time they promised your prescription would be ready.

She wondered how the place treated humans if this is how they dealt with the Creatures they thought were Very Special.

When she got to the counter.....

LASER LIGHT!!!!!! CHASE THE LASER!!!!!!

....she got the bad news. The slutty Persian sales rep had convinced the good veterinarian to start writing prescriptions for a hairball treatment that cost 20 times as much as anything else on the market, but had the clinical advantage of being advertised on TV. It would require a prior authorization from her insurance company. Spooky arched her back and stood her fur on end, but to no avail. She whipped out her cellphone and called the vet. The office was closed. She called the Drugmonkey. He was hung over and asleep. Spooky's tummy hurt. She coughed up a hairball on the counter and went home to mourn the wasted day.

Just Another Random Day At Work.

The first customer of the day slammed his vial on the counter. "THESE DON'T WORK!!" He semi-screamed. "ALL THEY DO IS MAKE ME PISS!"

The prescription was for furosemide.. Time for my counseling star to shine baby. The customer also had a prescription for Prozac that ordered me to "dispense 60 tablets by mouth" Maybe the act of me forming a nice little Prozac spitball then getting them to the patient like a mama bird was supposed to help snap him out of his depression. Anyway, after I puked Prozac all over him I explained that furosemide is a diuretic, which means that it does in fact make you piss a lot.

As this was going on a lady asked the high school kid mopping the cough/cold aisle where the Nasonex was. I watched them search the allergy section together for a good 10 minutes. Nasonex is prescription-only. I'm a bad man.

"Do you have any allergies to medicines?"

"You mean right now?"

A fax showed up from a doctor's office intended for the pharmacy on the other side of town. I forwarded it to its intended recipient and was rewarded for my good deed with a phone call a few minutes later:

"I'm not filling this! I can't be sure it really came from the doctor!!"

Good call. Because you really can't be too careful when you're dealing with ibuprofen prescriptions on a doctor's letterhead faxed to you from a licensed pharmacy. Like I've said, sometimes the customer is not the idiot.

"Hi, I'm calling from Dr. Dumbass' office with a prescription for a patient. Do you need the patients name?"

I decided I didn't, and just gave the pills she ordered to the next person who came up to the counter. Sometimes the customer isn't the idiot two times in a row.

"Is this the first time we've filled prescriptions for you?"
"Yes....oh....you mean today?"
Most of the time though, the customer is the idiot.

My technicians love the netflix. I don't know why. I never did hop on the netflix bandwagon This day my technicians were talking netflix yet again.....
"You have to see *No Country For Old Men*' next"
"They made a movie about Drugmonkey?"
Middle age approaches like a towering thundercloud on the horizon.....

The woman at the counter had tried to dress professionally but looked rather unnatural in her clothes. Go to any office park during lunch hour and you'll see no shortage of her type trying to powerwalk around the parking lot while wondering what Oprah would have eaten. "Is this the best thing to deal with stress?" she asked. She was holding a box of store-brand Ducolax, an over the counter medicine used for constipation.

I've learned the best thing to do in these situations is to get them talking. "What kind of stress are you dealing with exactly?" I said the words slowly, biding for time so I could think why on earth this woman thought she needed a stimulant laxative to deal with the burdens life was putting upon her.

"It's nothing in particular. I just need some help to relax sometimes so I can sleep."

Mystery solved. Relax. You see, the box of the store-brand Dulcolax was labeled only as "Corpo-pharmacy laxative"

Relax/laxative. Get it? Welcome to my world.

A Milestone In My Life. I Realize The Influence Of Larry "Bud" Melman Is Smaller Than That Of Even Ohio Northern University.

So the world is a small place my friends, and try try try as I might, the efforts I made to escape the one into which I was born will never be completely successful. This weekend I came across someone from Ada, Ohio. If you have ever heard of Ada, you know what that means. She was a college student. There are people who live in Ada who are not affiliated with Ohio Northern University, like 25 or so I think, and they are truly frightening individuals of such intellectual quality I doubt any of them could get piss out of a boot with instructions written on the heel. They make the footballs that are used by the National Football League. I'm not kidding about that.

But anyway, this woman did not make footballs, so naturally the small talk centered around Ohio Northern University, which was the institution that was foolish enough to grant me a degree in pharmacy. It went something like this....

Me: "Blah blah blah.....boring ONU small talk.......blah blah blah" Talk about ONU is unavoidably boring.

She: "Well we have a McDonald's now, after David Letterman mentioned on his show that we were the college campus furthest from one"

Me: "Really? We had Larry Bud Melman on campus once when I was there"

I was starting to perk up now. It had been a long time since I had thought of Larry Bud Melman and God I missed him.

Blank stare. Total blank stare. A blank stare that was the beginning of a shock I have yet to recover from.

"He was a regular on Letterman's show back when he was on at 12:30"

Incomprehension. I might as well have been speaking in tongues.

I walked back into the happy pill room slightly stunned. My keystone tech would help me out. My keystone tech always bails me out.

"Do you remember Larry Bud Melman?"

"Who?"

"You know who David Letterman is...."

"I think so.....the one who's not Jay Leno"

"You know he used to be on at 12:30"

"What?"

"You remember Johnny Carson....."

"Not really"

122

I looked around the store. Desperately. I mean, I know I'm getting old, but a lot of the stuff I liked when I wasn't old is still generally recognizable by the public. I just heard someone talking about fucking Fonzie the other day and Larry Bud Melman was better on his worst day than Fonzie ever was in his wet dreams. There was a time, my friends, when I would have been constantly surrounded by people hip to Larry Bud Melman, and now, as I looked around, I didn't see a soul I had any confidence would know the name. Larry has slipped off the earth and I failed to notice.

Or else Larry hasn't. I know I could put Larry Bud Melman into the Google, but if I do, and Larry isn't there, that means I'm not just old, but that I've gone insane. Toast on a stick. Melman Bus Lines. It might all be just in my head, and if it is, I can't take the risk of finding that out. This night I find myself quite possibly clinging to what could be the final facade of my sanity.

By the way, that wasn't a random expletive thrown in there in front of Fonzie. The person was actually talking about having sex with the former sitcom icon.

At least in my head they were. I think.

I Never Thought I Would Miss The Weather Report.

Especially since there really isn't any weather in California. It gets a little warmer, it gets a little cooler, sometimes it rains. That's the extent of the weather in my part of California. For awhile though, almost every night at work, I got a report that "It's a little cool out there." At first I admit I found it annoying. I find almost everyone annoying. Night after night though, the little old man in the 1930's style cap shuffling around the shopping center to get his exercise wore me down. He knew the way to get to me was to give me an opportunity to bitch about work.

"Looks like you're awful busy, but at least you got an inside job. It's a little cool out there tonight."

I think the first words I might have said to him were "You got the busy part right" He took that little crack in the Drugmonkey toughguy act and used it to drive a wedge through my wall against the outside world. The chats gradually got a little longer. One time I saw him coming up the aisle with a big old smile on his face. He opened up his outer coat to show me his original letter jacket from high school. I admit he looked so cute I just burst out laughing. It was a little cool out that night.

I learned he was in his 90's

He was born in the town where I work and had lived there his whole life.

He used to run track. That's where the letter jacket came from.

I never saw him with anyone else.

I never saw him get a prescription.

I never knew his name.

And one night I realized I haven't seen him in a few days. Crap. It doesn't take my Mensa card to figure out what happened. That jacket is most likely headed to one of the thrift shops on the other side of town. And no matter what I do in the next 40 years or so, I will end up in the exact same place. I'm not saying I'll end up in the thrift shop. That'd be kinda gross. You know what I mean. Ashes to ashes.

So why am I gonna schlep off to the pillbox of sweat tomorrow like a good little boy? Why don't I just stay up all night jamming tunes too loud, pack up my car and head to the Grand Canyon in the morning? I'd like to see the Grand Canyon. You know I've never smoked weed? Seriously, not once. Why not? Am I afraid of some father of the skies keeping a ledger on my life's rights and wrongs? Um, no. I'm an atheist. So why exactly don't I just empty out my bank account on a few high class hookers and a couple laps around the world? Why get close to anyone at all? You'll still end up just as alone.

The same pile of ashes. I would be better off if I had just growled at that old man the first time I saw him.

Other than AIDS. That would be a good reason to avoid the escorts, but I think you get my point.

It's not as cool tonight as it usually is.

I have no idea why I ever got into this profession.

Fucking plastic motorcycle.

Dear Insurance Company, And Seemingly Every Other Company That Runs A Call Center.

Here's a fucking idea Einsteins.

Instead of suggesting that I am taxing your poor little delicate corporate soul by daring to call for assistance during what you say is one of your "peak hours," how about maybe.....and this may sound a little radical for you so hang with me here.....

....scheduling more of your employees to work during these peak hours, in order to be better able to handle the increased number of calls you know you will receive? I know it sounds like crazy talk, but your whole business was built upon the assumption that health care providers would be eager to sign contracts that would pay them less money than they were currently making, which must have sounded pretty crazy itself back in the day.

I mean, it's no secret when these peak hours are. You've already figured them out and don't hesitate to tell me while I am on hold. Endlessly on hold.

You may wonder where this stroke of out of the box thinking came from, where a train of thought so fundamentally different from the thoughts used to guide your decisions until now could have possibly originated. I'll be happy to share. It came to me when I asked myself what my customers would say to me if I said that maybe they should come back during one of my "non peak hours." They'd tell me to fuck off and die, that's what they'd do.

So I guess I'm just a little confused as to why you shouldn't fuck off and die as well.

And by the way, if you are constantly experiencing "call volume that is heavier than normal" it may be time to re-adjust your definition of normal.

Just sayin'

Fuckers.

Another Quick Question For My Friends In The Insurance Industry

If you can print off a letter that says someone is covered, and that their card containing all the info needed to file a claim on their behalf is on the way, and that while this letter doesn't contain a scrap of information your pharmacist will need to file any claims, you should bring it to the store with you and wave it around like a lunatic anyway.....

Is there some reason.....you couldn't take the time and resources that you used to print and mail this useless letter and do something like.....

......oh I dunno.....maybe......

PRINT THE ACTUAL FUCKING CARD?.......AND MAIL THE ACTUAL FUCKING CARD? THE SAME WAY YOU MAILED THIS GODDAMN LETTER????

Call me crazy, but I'm thinking it could be done. Some nights just lend themselves to big dreams I guess.

But It Was The New Very Berry Flavor. Surely That Works Better.

The perps knew exactly what they were doing. The lighting in the video was dark and foreboding, yet the two days worth of facial stubble on the face of the hostage came through just as clearly as the desperation contained behind his fearful eyes.

"I am a fraud, and I'm sorry it ever came to this," the voice softly cracked into the camera. "I just want to say I miss my wife and family very much, and I hope you listen to the requests of my captors"

The knife pressed against his throat as the screen went dark.

A week ago it had all seemed so easy. A week ago he was making a routine presentation to another health department strapped for cash and feeling overwhelmed and overstressed. He knew their budget had been cut. He knew health departments did not like the expense of fighting off infections. A full-scale deployment of the immune system was not cheap. And he knew most health departments were run by the brain cells that were not exactly the sharpest knives in the drawer.

He was Airborne, and he had made a pretty good living off people who can't understand the words "there is no cure for the common cold"

This time, however, he was up against the flu, or possibly Pneumococcal pneumonia.

He knew something was wrong as soon as he merged into the bloodstream. His plan was to check into his hotel and lay low for a week, then emerge and claim all credit and a fat paycheck when the cold had resolved itself, the way it always does. The blood was warm though. Too warm. Broken white blood cells were lying in the median, some crying, some too exhausted to move, some on the verge of death. "The doxycycline......oh God....the doxycycline is here....we might have a chance" muttered the shell-shocked white blood cell lieutenant. Airborne had no idea what he was talking about and slowly drove past. He heard the unique laughter that marks the mentally broken as he pulled away, but he knew it was too late to turn back.

That night five armed intruders broke into his hotel room, and they did terrible things to Airborne. They found orifices he had no idea were there. They created new orifices. They gave him pain like he never experienced in his wildest nightmares. They made him say it as they chopped off one of his fingers:

"The Airborne health formula helps to support your immune system through its blend of vitamins and minerals. Airborne's unique combination of vitamins, nutrients and proprietary blend of herbal extracts all work together to create the formula people swear by."

They laughed and made him say it again and chugged more tequila. Then they cut off another one of his fingers and made the video where he begged for his life.

Doxycycline found what was left of Airborne's corpse as soon as he emerged through the duodenum. He winced, but did not weep. In the end, no one wept for Airborne. The wife he claimed to miss so much spent the life insurance settlement on breast enhancement surgery, and Airborne was buried in an unmarked grave, along with the hopes of a million or so suckers who thought there was a cure for the common cold.

Doxycycline met up with members of the white blood cell patrol and the warmth of overheated blood surrounded them the way a swarm of old people surround a pharmacy gate five minutes before it's scheduled to open. Surrounded just a little too much, thought doxyxycline as they cleared the capillary pass and started to merge onto the vein highway. The white blood cell captain knew there would be trouble. It was just way too warm.

"We might have to go into the lymph" He told the rest of the patrol. This captain could sense trouble the way a cat can sense that it should poop only in the littlerbox.

Two hours later they found it. Or rather, the confused private found it. Six months ago he was a stem cell back in the marrow and looked out over a future of limitless opportunities. He decided to join The White Blood Cell Corps because he thought it would be a good way to get out and see the body. He also needed money to get into Nerve Cell University. He wanted to study music, but now he had a protein shell in his hands.

"What is it Capt'n?"

"I was afraid of this, but I didn't want to scare you men. The viruses are shedding. We're gonna have a fight on our hands."

A stunned silence washed over the patrol. The Captain was the only one who could remember the last viral war. "Don't worry men. It won't be anything we can't handle. Just pray to your momma the bacteria don't get involved though. Things get ugly when the bacteria get involved."

The first skirmish didn't go well. To the boy from Marrow it seemed almost as if the viruses were manufacturing themselves faster than they could be killed. The Captain said later that's exactly what they do. They hijack innocent cells and manufacture themselves.

"Don't worry son. The antibodies are on the way. If it's just a fight with the viruses the antibodies will be all we need"

The boy was afraid to ask, but the Captain knew what was on his mind. "You have to be ready for the bacteria son. Surrounding these little specks of zombie protein is nothing compared to eating a bacteria alive. You have to be ready for that."

The boy started to weep softly.

"Pray the bacteria do not come." Said doxycycline as he lit his last cigarette. "I'll stop their protein synthesis all right. But just pray it doesn't come to that."

They heard a soft rustling in the woods.

His Was Not To Question Why.....

He struggled to get the proper grip around the Xanax. He wasn't sure if he could handle it. He wasn't sure he wanted to handle it. But the Xanax was there. And there were needs for the Xanax.

Upward he went. Higher and higher. Above and away from the day to day minutia of the world, thinking only of the Xanax. How did it come to this point? Why was he doing this? The Xanax seemed to weigh him down as if he were carrying the entire universe beneath him. He thought about letting go and drifting towards the light.

He loved the light, but instead he beat his wings a little harder and carried on. He hoped a bat did not get him.

After what seemed like five eternities he was able to let go. To release himself from the burdens the Xanax had put upon him. He dropped it into the warm, wet cavern of darkness where it belonged and tried not to be overwhelmed by the stench of the person's recently eaten dinner. Garlic.....he was thankful he was not a vampire. Mission accomplished, the Xanax released, he went off to flutter towards the light, for he had earned it.

Two more times and he could call it a day.

At least that's how I imagined it as I looked at the label from the drugstore on the other side of town and its instructions: to "Take 1 tablet by moth three times a day" That's actually not too bad for those guys.

I dialed the phone to begin the transfer and settled in for what I knew would be a long wait.

Perhaps I Should Have Taken That Communications Elective In College.

I realized that day I had been behind the pharmacy counter 15 years. My life was drifting down the chute like sand in an hourglass and I still couldn't tell you why I ever picked this profession. I woke up that morning and felt another grey hair come in. Old age loomed on the horizon and I still had no idea why I had made the biggest decision of my life.

There was no turning back though. I was now an experienced pharmacist.

I have to admit experience has its advantages though. I take great pride in the ability I've developed over the years of answering pointless, meandering, substance-free questions with responses of equal quality. Don't get me wrong, real questions always get real answers, but there is such a thing as a stupid question. Everyone in the profession knows it, and I've had enough practice with them that I have perfected the art of the non-offensive blowoff. Or so I thought until tonight.

It started off normally enough. Middle aged non-retarded looking dude tells the tech he wants to talk to the pharmacist. Fine. Tech let's me know and I walk over. The guy is holding a box of nicotine patches in his hand. This is the entirety of his statement to me, complete and unedited:

"STEP ONE"

It was said in such a way that I don't know whether to put a question mark or an exclamation point at the end of the quote.

I waited for more. There was no more. I had no idea what to say to this fuck. He had a look of expectation on his face. Finally I said:

"Yup, that's step one. Just like it says on the box"

The man looked at me for a bit then walked off in a huff like he was convinced he had just talked to the stupidest person in the world.

I'm still not sure what this guy was expecting. I am still sure though, that I am perfectly capable of answering a question if you are capable of forming one.

A Story Of Unparalled Customer Service. In Your Face Wal-Mart

I had been getting the living piss beat out of me for about nine and a half hours when the phone rang. This is the unedited beginning of the conversation:

Me: Thank you for calling corpo-pharmacy, may I help you?

Dumbass: IS THERE A (name of corpo pharmacy chain here) OFF THE LAWRENCE EXPRESSWAY??

Here is a summary of my thoughts over the next two seconds:

Well hello to you too.

There is one highway in this little town. Its name isn't Lawrence.

The nearest city that is big enough to name its highways would be about 80 miles away.

There is no guarantee that is the city this person is talking about.

Fuck this guy.

"Yeah, you take the first exit after the big overpass, make a right at the light, and it's in the strip center with the McDonalds." Is what I said. Or something like that. I don't remember exactly, as it was a totally random set of directions for a city that existed only in my mind. If I had been given the name of a real city maybe I would have done better.

The sound the dumbass made before he hung up the phone was something like..."hhhuuurroookk"

I immediately felt bad. What if I just steered some prissy-ass white boy into the ghetto and a carjacking? What if he was trying to get a prescription filled for a kid who didn't know Daddy was both extremely dumb and extremely rude? Crap. Maybe this time the Drugmonkey had gone too far.

Another call about 10 minutes later. "YEAH, I'M AT THE COUNTER HERE AND THIS PHARMACIST SAYS THEY DON'T HAVE MY INSURANCE ON FILE."

He found it. The dumbass fucking found it. I think the key was my mentioning of the McDonalds. "Take a right and look for the McDonalds" just might work in any situation really. I wondered if Burger King might be the key to getting the guy's insurance card to work.

I suppose I could use Google to find out where the Lawrence Expressway is, but at this point I really don't want to know. I hate all people.

An Interview With Governor George Wallace.

George Wallace, called "the most influential loser in 20th century politics" by biographer Dan Carter, first gained notional notoriety in 1963 when, as Governor, he made a famous "stand in the schoolhouse door," as a show of defiance to federal orders to desegregate the University of Alabama. Starting with his inauguration earlier that year, where he famously declared "segregation today . . . segregation tomorrow . . . segregation forever," Wallace practiced the politics of racial division throughout his rise to prominence, running what Carter called "one of the most racist campaigns in modern southern political history" in seeking re-election to the Governor's office in 1970.

Wallace ran for President four times, carrying five states in 1968 and coming close to his goal of throwing the election into the House of Representatives, where he had hoped to use his status as a power broker to end federal efforts at desegregation. Four years later he was shot on the campaign trail while again seeking the Presidency, leaving him paralyzed for the remainder of his life.

He later renounced his segregationist views and served two more terms as Alabama's Governor, leaving office in 1987. The Drugmonkey caught up with Wallace in the fourth level of hell, where he has resided since his death in 1998.

DM- Thank you for taking the time to speak with me Governor Wallace, I'm sure you're a busy man.

Wallace- EEEYYYAAAGAGAHHHHHH!!!!! THE POWER OF BEEZEBUB IS UNQUESTIONED!!!! WHHOOOOOGGGHHHHH!!!... I'm sorry about that son, demons and all down here, I'm sure you understand.

DM- Certainly. I wonder if you've had much of a chance to stay in touch with what's happening in American politics during your time in hell.

W- Oh absolutely. I dedicated my life on planet earth to the art of politics and they've been kind enough here to allow me to keep up in between burnings of my naked body in boiling oil.

DM- So naturally my first question is your reaction to the election of President Obama.

W- It's hard to believe isn't it? "I mean, you got the first mainstream African-American who is articulate and bright and clean and a nice-looking guy, I mean, that's a storybook, man. I think his success comes, in part, from his light-skinned appearance and speaking patterns with no Negro dialect, unless he wants to have one."*

DM- It almost seems like the modern "Tea Party" movement has taken a few pages from the old Wallace Presidential playbook.

W- Son, there's nothing modern about those Tea Partiers. Talk of the 10th Amendment and states rights? Racist fear-based demagoguery manipulating the white working class? Setting up the federal government as a bogyman punching bag? My God I was doing all that almost 50 years ago. The main difference is in my day all we had was the Jew-controlled, Communist-lovin' media. If I woulda had me Sean Hannity and those boys over at Fox News, let me tell you I would have been wrapping up my second term in the White House right in time for the bicentennial.

Please excuse the swarm of locusts that just came from my eyes.

DM- Did you ever see the assassination attempt that left you in constant pain for the last 26 years of your life as the work of Karma?

W- What? No, the boy that shot me's name was Bremer

DM- Yes, but maybe that it was part of a larger cosmic force set in motion by some of the things you'd done in politics?

W- No, that boy was just crazy, they found his dairy, and he said he was just looking to be famous. He was either gonna shoot me or Nixon.

DM- I see. Governor, why do you think you ended up down here, even after you renounced your segregationist views and said of your stand in the schoolhouse door, "I was wrong. Those days are over and they ought to be over."

W- I've thought about that son, and you know, it's easy to look back and do the right thing. The apology of a broken old man doesn't count for a whole lot. When it mattered, I was worse than silent. I rode a river of hate because I thought it would make me a great man, but what I became was a piece of dirt in the dustbin of history. Now all I am is a lesson. To those who choose to listen.

Wallace then cried tears of fire, which seared the flesh of his face.

This quote is a combination of things actually said by Joe Biden and Harry Reid

The Makers Of Kaopectate Need To Have The Crap Beat Out Of Them.

Kaopectate is effective at relieving diarrhea.
Kaopectate generally produces a bowel movement in 12 to 72 hours.
Kaopectate can be taken to relieve diarrhea cause by antibiotic use.
Kaopectate is not recommended for diarrhea caused by antibiotic use.

I have not lied to you. I can say these things because the asswipes that own the Kaopectate brand name, Chattem, Inc., have taken the original Kaopectate formula containing attapulgite, which we all knew and loved as the only product to be used for antibiotic-induced diarrhea, and changed it to bismuth subsalicylate, the same ingredient found in Pepto Bismol. Bismuth subsalicylate is not recommended for relief of antibiotic induced diarrhea. It also should not be given to children with viral infections, which will be no source of confusion to people who remember the old "Children's Kaopectate" brand.

Wait, there's more. The caring professionals at Chattem have also decided to change the name of Surfak, a stool softening laxative to........Kaopectate.

So....Kaopectate makes you poop, and Kaopectate stops you from pooping. Clear as mud isn't it?

To be fair, Chattem isn't the only company that does this kind of marketing bullshit.

Maalox is Pepto Bismol as well. Except when it's just regular Maalox.

Remember, you can't give Pepto Bismol to children. Unless it's children's Pepto, which is only an antacid, unlike Pepto Bismol, which works as an anti-nausea and anti-diarrheal as well. Proctor & Gamble chose to make this distinction clear by using the same color scheme and font for both Children's Pepto and Pepto Bismol, which are, again, two entirely different products. That's why the labels look almost exactly the same. And they both use the word "Pepto." Because they're different.

Tylenol is also Benadryl, which is also Nytol.

Midol is Tylenol with a dash of caffeine, except when Midol is Advil, or when Midol is Aleve.

Neosporin is Micatin, an effective athlete's foot remedy. Except when it's Neosporin the first aid ointment, which is totally ineffective against athlete's foot.

Now you know why your pharmacist has no interest in hearing any questions about "Tylenol" or "Maalox" or "Kaopectate" when you're asking about over the counter products. The first thing they'll do is flip the box over and look for the part of the label that lists the active ingredient. Because Tylenol is Midol and Midol is Aleve. Except when Tylenol is Benadryl.

I could go on all day, but I prefer the simplicity of scotch, which is just scotch.

This One's For My Southern Baptist Friends, Who Make Up A Big Chunk Of The One-Third Of Americans Who Believe The Bible Is The Word Of God To Be Taken Literally

"And as for thy bondmen, and thy bondmaids, whom thou shalt have; of the nations that are round about you, of them shall ye buy bondmen and bondmaids." -Leviticus 25:44

My Canadian slave's name is Ian. I've owned him for about five years now.

I remember thinking when I was born again that Vancouver would be a good place to shop for slaves. I love Vancouver, and I bought a small wooden totem pole sculpture there once that is absolutely beautiful. But then I realized that that fair city probably has the mildest climate and most cosmopolitan atmosphere in any of the provinces, which would mean that any slaves from there would probably be soft and weak. I wanted a slave from a place where life was a little tougher. Where nature and nurture would throw some character-building adversity into its residents. I also wanted a major airport though, because I thought the quicker I could get my slave away from Canada and into God's chosen land the better. I decided on Edmonton.

I saw Ian standing next to the cash register at the Eddie Bauer store in the Kingsway Mall. There's an old joke that the quickest way to get a roomful of Canadians to shut up is to say something like "please be quiet," so I looked at Ian and said "please follow me," and like a good Canadian, he did. That must be why God wants you to get your slaves from neighboring countries, so you don't have to mess with nets and whips and slave ships like when we got our slaves from Africa. I left $50 next to the cash register, but then realized that the onerous tax rates that Canadians must bear in order to finance their public health system would probably push Ian's final price to something like $75. Fucking socialists. I still thought I got a pretty good bargain though. Ian seemed like a strapping young lad, and was very obedient from the start.

It wasn't long though until I had a few second thoughts. Ian didn't seem to work nearly as hard as the Mexican slaves most of my friends had. I remember thinking that those Catholics south of the border wouldn't understand the covenant between man and God that the Holy Bible represents, being members of the Papist cult that they are. But boy, was I wrong. Every morning my neighbor's Mexican slaves would be up at the crack of dawn, mowing the yard, cleaning the house, cooking breakfast, when it was all I could do to get Ian to wake up at noon, which only gave him two hours to get the condo ready for me when I got up. He was totally useless during the Stanley Cup finals, and I suspect he reveres Queen Elizabeth more than the prophet of God George W. Bush himself. The only thing he really turned out to be good for was running over to the liquor store to get more scotch.

Which after many months of prayer I realized was the only thing I needed a slave for anyway. I've scoured Leviticus and the rest of God's book and I don't see anything there about any specific work your bondman is supposed to do, so I guess as long as I acquired him from a nation that is around me that makes it right with the Lord.

I still might put in a bid for my neighbor's Pedro though.

A Random Tribute To Pete Seeger

If your musical taste has never gone beyond the modern music machine that gives us American Idol and Lady Gaga, you're probably not a fan of folk music, and you may never have heard of Pete Seeger, which would be a shame for you. Pete is simultaneously the greatest voice and last echo of the working man's folk music of the Great Depression, a last reminder of the time when *This Land Is Your Land* had all its verses.

"What are you talking about Drugmonkey? *This Land Is Your Land*? I've heard that song a million times"

But you probably haven't heard all of it. You've heard the sanitized version. The homogenized remnant that has been processed into mindless rah rah pap to be played on Disneyland's Main Street USA as Mickey Mouse walks by. The original was in your face political. A song of the working man who wasn't going to take being exploited by this country's self appointed economic elite much longer.

> *As I went walking I saw a sign there*
> *And on the sign it said "No Trespassing."*
> *But on the other side it didn't say nothing,*
> *That side was made for you and me.*

> *Nobody living can ever stop me,*
> *As I go walking that freedom highway;*
> *Nobody living can ever make me turn back*
> *This land was made for you and me.*

> *In the squares of the city, In the shadow of a steeple;*
> *By the relief office, I'd seen my people.*
> *As they stood there hungry, I stood there asking,*
> *Is this land made for you and me?*

That's how Woody Guthrie wrote it, and that's how Pete Seeger sings it to this day. An unapologetic leftist, he was blacklisted at the height of his group's popularity and dragged in front of Congress to testify before the

House Un-American Activities committee, where he was asked about his past ties to Communists and pressured to name names of fellow travelers. Here's what Pete said:

> "I am not going to answer any questions as to my association, my philosophical or religious beliefs or my political beliefs, or how I voted in any election, or any of these private affairs. I think these are very improper questions for any American to be asked, especially under such compulsion as this."

With those words Pete Seeger's music career had the knees knocked out from under it, and he was indicted for contempt of Congress. I'll leave it to you to decide which side was Un-American that day.

Pete spent the better part of the next decade in the wilderness, his ability to earn a living crippled while fighting a legal battle that at one point resulted in a sentence, later overturned, of 10 years in a federal prison. It took The Smothers Brothers to reintroduce Pete to a mass audience.

Yes. Those Smothers Brothers. They had a variety show during the 60's and fought a tooth and nail battle with CBS to have Pete on. While the existence of testicles on The Smothers Brothers may come as a surprise to those who see them today, there is no doubt Pete has an iron pair. At a time when it had not yet become fashionable to protest the Vietnam War, Pete got on national television after an exile imposed by the United States Congress and sang *Waist Deep In The Big Muddy* to Mr. and Mrs. America:

"We were lucky to escape from the Big Muddy/When the big fool said to push on..."

Kick-ass. Not to mention depressingly familiar.

Oh, and along the way, Pete Seeger formed Hudson River Sloop Clearwater, an organization that convinced people the Hudson River was crazy polluted and should be cleaned up.

I saw Pete Seeger not long ago. When I heard he was coming close I knew I would have crawled through mud and ice and snow and rain on my knees for miles for the chance to see him. Fortunately all I had to do was buy a ticket. He was 90 years old, and he held that arena in the absolute palm of his hand. I wanted to wrap myself around him and make him stay forever, as I fear they just don't make his kind anymore. The fact I couldn't made me want to cry a little, along with the continued power of the songs I heard that day.

Pete won't be with us much longer. If he comes to your town I recommend crawling on your hands and knees to see him if you have to.

And don't ever forget the lost verses.

Another Random Day Of Pill Counting Highlights

It's never easy to hear tales of woe and agony, much less witness them firsthand. But the human condition is such that we all face obstacles we must try to overcome. The challenges life throws our way will not always be fair, but we have no choice to struggle on. Struggle in pursuit of the hope that someday, if not for us, karma or our creator will smile upon our actions in some way that will benefit the cosmic force that governs life. We struggle, but often unsuccessfully, and while it is not pleasurable to watch, I knew what I was getting into when I picked my profession. I was reminded of this as I walked through the door to begin my workday.

"OH COME ON!!!!! I SLID MY CARD ALREADY" The woman said as I got ready to assume the position, and my heart broke for the old wrinkly bitch. The way she summoned up the strength and quiet dignity to slide her American Express through the credit card reader again, when by all rights she should not have had to, inspired me to move forward in the struggles of my own life.

The first call I took was from a woman who wanted to know the time. She calls often and says she's blind and needs to know when to take her medication. For some reason I don't fuck with her, maybe because she does manage to tie in her insanity with pharmaceutical care, unlike a good portion of the wackjobs who get past my employer's voice mail. I did finally realize today though, that the woman takes her meds four times a day, and the store closes every night for 12 hours. I think she may be using me.

The next call I took was from a customer who wanted to know if their prescription had any refills.

"I don't see where we've ever filled that for you ma'am"

"Oh, you've never filled it, I get it through mail order. So do I have any refills left?"

I remembered the inspiration of the lady at the credit card machine and vowed to struggle on.

From the front register I received a report that someone demanded to exchange an empty box of dental floss for a new one. "It fell out, it was defective!" they said. They had also spit in it. That's why you stay in school kids, because when you're behind the drug counter wearing a white coat you don't have to be nearly as nice to people like that as that poor schlep up front had to be. You will, however, have to nervously do mathematical calculations upon receiving a prescription for 26.25ml of cefinidir and breathe a sigh of relief upon realizing that the physician's assistant absolutely walked the perfect line between the minimum effective dose of 26.24ml and 26.26ml, which would have been instantly fatal.

A person tried to pick up a prescription for their uncle who had died. Vicodin. Surprise!

As I made my exit through the store's front door to end this day's commitment to my employer, I saw the poor schlep who had to deal with the dental floss incident chase down a teenage girl.

"Ma'am.....you forgot your cash back!!"

"What? I get cash back? Wow! I didn't know that!!"

There you go, sometimes the karma of the credit card reader taketh away, but sometimes it giveth as well.

An Open Letter To My Old Boss.

Hiya boss,

   You may be surprised to be hearing from me. I know it's been awhile, and the last words we shared weren't exactly filled with happy thoughts, but I thought of you today and thought I'd drop you a line. You see, about an hour before closing time tonight I had to call one of your stores for a prescription transfer. Being on hold for 20 minutes before speaking to a clerk for 10 seconds who put me back on hold for 10 minutes to speak to the pharmacist really brought back the memories. I always wonder when I'm in a holdfest like this, which I am a couple times a week, what would happen if I were a customer calling to ask if it's a problem that my grandma accidentally took a couple extra doses of amitriptyline. Not that you or any of your ilk give a rat's ass about anyone's grandma. The only thing that gets your willy hard is the thought of more prescriptions flowing through your place at a lower cost to fill per unit. That's why you were so overjoyed when your chain bought out the last independent pharmacy in town and added 25% to our workload literally overnight. The day you told us we could have one extra tech to handle the 300 extra prescriptions a day your deal would mean for us was the only time I ever saw you smile. Good times. Remember the time the 18 month old girl got the nitroglycerin pills intended for an 87 year old man? Boy, I sure do. The only thing worse than making a mistake on a prescription is dealing with the fallout from a prescription mistake that you DIDN'T make. Did I ever tell you why your drawer was short that day? You see, the parent of the child who could have died wanted the money refunded that they spent for the pills that could have ended their daughter's life. Fair enough. So, I followed your company policy and paged a member of management. I always thought it was a bit odd how you had no problem leaving me alone all night in a room with a couple thousand OxyContin, but thought it necessary to have a community college dropout be the one to return fourteen dollars and ninety-nine cents, but hey, you write the paychecks. The customer whose child could have died didn't see it that way though, and was about ready to kill someone himself by the time we paged the dropout for the third time. That's when I opened the drawer, handed the man whose child could have died two twenty dollar bills and told him I was sorry how this whole thing went down from beginning to end. That the customer saw I was breaking your pointless policy for him was probably the only thing that prevented a lawsuit. You're welcome.

I wonder if you remember our discussion afterwards of what happened. Probably not, because you really didn't even seem to hear a word I was saying at the time. I told you how that store was breaking its employees and endangering the public. That your company was woefully negligent and it was only a matter of time before someone would hold the place to account. I asked you what your plan was to improve things. You said.....you'd give me $30,000 not to quit, thereby missing entirely the point of me threatening to leave in the first place. With that money you could have hired another full time employee, but you thought the best way to keep someone else's child, mother, or grandfather out of danger was to throw some Benjamin's into my bank account and keep everything the same. I know it's physically impossible to fuck yourself, but I don't regret telling you to do so.

I hear not much has changed for you or your company, but things are much better for me now. I have a new job in a store that does about a quarter the prescription volume of your place, a store that's considered to be a laggard in its district. You see, my new boss, he's no different from you. The only thing keeping him from running me and the rest of the staff into the ground is the company's inability to drum up enough business to do so. Stockholders are angry, but the people who do come in the door are well taken care of, the exact opposite of the stockholder/customer relationship at your place. Funny how that works. I'll let you get back to work now. I know you have important things to do, like maybe meeting with the corporate lawyer to discuss how much is a fair price to offer the parents of a dead child.

Just make sure to get a confidentiality agreement. You don't want the stock price adversely affected.

Sincerely,

Drugmonkey

Somewhere Along The Way A Piece Of Me Was Liberated. I Know Not When.

I will attempt in this chapter to describe to you the grip that college football has on most of the state of Ohio. I will fail. Unless you were born there, or someplace like Michigan, Nebraska, Oklahoma, or Alabama, places so empty of culture and possibilities for a meaningful life that the whole of a persons physical and spiritual existence is manifested through a game where boys play fight over a leather air-filled sack, you don't and never will know what it is like to be born into the cult of the poisonous nut. My mother is a little old lady who can always tell you the score of last week's game. I visited my sister once in Columbus, home of the University of the Poisonous Nut, during the weekend of the annual game with their hated rivals, the Michigan Weasel Cousins. Every time the Poisonous Nuts scored a point, the entire building literally shook. I had a drink knocked off her coffee table.

That building may have collapsed in 2006. Those of you who follow sports may know what I'm talking about. The Poisonous Nuts and the Weasel Cousins were the number 1 and 2 ranked teams in college football, and they met to fight over that leather sack. I dreaded the day, for I knew that I would have to watch. Even though I had long ago escaped to the coast, I knew that just as the Eagles once sang about the Hotel California, you can check out of the Poisonous Nut cult anytime you like, but you can never leave. A few years earlier the Poisonous Nuts played the Miami Weather Disturbances for the national college football championship. I was working, so I taped the game. I am ashamed of this. I am more ashamed that I was watching the tape at 2 in the morning shouting things like TACKLE HIM! GODDAMMIT, TACKLE THAT SON OF A BITCH! Any illusions that I was a sophisticated, classy, intellectual type of guy went right out my lungs that night, and I knew that from then on, the best I could do would be to try and hide this flaw of character.

So that afternoon, as my cult masters readied to take the field to battle Emmanuel Goldstein in the three hours of hate, I pulled the curtains closed and turned on the television, resigned to my fate. What happened though, was that I saw only a bunch of straight boys who don't realize they're gay dressed in panty hose hitting each other really hard for no apparent reason. It really was a good game if you're into that kind of thing, close, hard fought....put in your favorite sports cliché here. But the only time I got emotional witnessing the spectacle was when I found a bag of the good salsa chips in the back of my cupboard.

I know most of you don't realize what this means. It means that this...thing...it wasn't in my genes, I'm not an animal....I'm......I'm.....

Free. Gloriously free....

So as the celebratory riots were certainly underway in Columbus, I stood that night born into a new world. A wonderful world where affection between men doesn't have to be limited to public play-fight rituals. You are free to love each other however you choose men of my world!

But not to love me.....I still like boobs. Just wanna be clear on that.

The Melatonin Chronicles.....Or, Bizzaro Dream #2

The bizzaro dream is coming, I promise, but first the necessary background:

Detroit was ground zero for the dark, seething underbelly of the 60's. Everybody remembers the happy hippies of Woodstock, but we have tried to forget the very real anger that was just as much a part of that era. While the flower children were doing their thing, singing how we should just smile on our brother and learn to love one another right now, Detroit bands like The Stooges and MC5 were letting us know what it was like to have your teeth kicked in by the cops and then be charged with assault. My kind of music. Now I love the MC5, but I hadn't been listening to them much lately. You know how it is; music works its way to the back of your collection for awhile, only to be re-discovered years later. That night, however, the MC5 came back into my life as I slept.

In my dream, I had decided that it was time for me to learn to play the bass guitar, and so I had signed up for some classes at the local community college. The instructor enters the classroom, and it is none other than the bass player for the MC5. Sweet! I will finally be able to ask him about the jar!

"Um...the jar?" I hear you saying. You see, the first MC5 album I bought years ago had a rather, um....disturbing picture on the back. It featured one of the band members, with a giant afro, looking disturbed and/or high, holding a large jar and pointing at it with his other hand.

That jar has fascinated me from the day I first laid eyes on it. What could possibly be inside? Would I really want to know? The way the dude with the afro was pointing at it it almost looked like he was soliciting spare change so he can take the bus home after the gig. In my dream though, the mystery of the jar was about to be solved! I sat patiently through class, barely able to concentrate on the lesson knowing that this obsession of mine was about to be put to rest. After class, as I made my way up to the front of the room my heart rate quickened with anticipation........

Then I woke up. And my heart really was beating fast. Why the hell would my brain be thinking in the middle of the night about a band I haven't consciously thought of in years? Why would the mystery of the jar surface now after lying dormant for so long? DAMN YOU JAR! I WILL UNLOCK YOUR SECRET SOMEDAY!

I'm thinking I should talk to my doctor about Ambien, and, um, maybe a few other things.

Thanks To The DEA, I Now Have The World's Longest Schlong, And One Of The Thickest.

This realization came in that day's mail. Mixed in with the usual advertisements for Wonderpill XR™ and corporate sponsored continuing education was the store's self certification certificate from the Drug Enforcement Administration. Yes, a "self certification certificate" was exactly as stupid as it sounds. It works like this:

1) The government issues new regulations regarding the sale of pseudoephedrine, the nasal decongestant you've known and loved for years as Sudafed. If you've had a cold in the last few years, or if you make a lot of crystal meth, you know exactly what I'm talking about. You can't buy Sudafed and friends anymore without signing for it, showing some ID, and saying "Lloyd Duplantis of Gray, Louisiana is not worthy to act as my decongestant by sucking the mucus out of my sinuses." The third requirement just applies to my store, when I'm working and in the right mood. More about Lloyd Duplantis later in the book.

2) The government then makes pharmacies promise to be good and obey the new regulations.

3) Pharmacies then get a certificate saying they are complying with the law.

A kicker is that at one time the DEA was planning on charging a $35 fee for issuance of this certificate. I shit you not. The government was going to charge money for the privilege of obeying the law. I don't know if the fee went through as planned. One of many benefits of not being the pharmacy manager is that I don't have to give a shit about such details.

So this is what it's come to my friends. In 40 years we've gone from Ralph Nader taking down General Motors for selling coffins on wheels to businesses "complying" with the law by saying that they are. In the spirit of this new era of corporate regulation I would like to issue the following self-certification. My wiener is 24 inches long, and at least 100% thicker than the average male's. I will be happy to provide a certificate certifying the accuracy of these statements. Just drop me an e-mail.

Friday Night Freak....

God I miss the ghetto sometimes. Working in the ghetto a book can just write itself, all I had to do is take a few notes.......

Short little dude comes to the counter and asks if we have his medicine. I swear the only difference between him and the oompa loompa men from Willy Wonka is that the customer is white and not orange. I tell oompa that there is nothing ready and he walks away confused. This type of thing only happens about seven thousand times during the course of an average workday. Oompa returns about an hour later to check again.

Me: "There's still nothing here for you sir. What medicine did you need?"
Oompa: "Cannabis"
Me: "Excuse me?"
Oompa: "Here, this should explain everything"
Oopma then hands me a picture of his mug shot and booking info from the county jail.

Me: "I gotta be honest sir. This doesn't explain anything. Was your doctor going to phone in a prescription for you? "
Oompa: "They told me the cannabis would be here."
Me: "Who told you the cannabis would be here?"
Oompa then drifts away from the counter like a ship cut away from its anchor. I saw him awhile later in the snack aisle. Snacking probably just isn't the same without your cannabis.

The only theory I can come up with is that a corrupt cop or fellow prisoner duped Oompa out of his stash upon his entry into the correctional system and told him as part of the ruse that it would be stored for safekeeping at my pharmacy. If that is the case I would say only that there was no need to keep me out of the loop. Just clue me in next time guys, and I'll be happy to fuck with his little Oompa brain some more when he's at the counter. I might even sing a little.

Ommpa...loompa....doompadee doo....
I've got a perfect puzzle for you......

My secret plan to win the Nobel Prize In Medicine....

Ok....so before I spring the Nobel secret on you, I'll have to give you some background information. My little plot will end up ridding the world of tuberculosis, the respiratory infection that has plagued humankind since probably close to the time people began to breathe. TB is treatable today, for the most part. The problem is, you'll have to take a combination of antibiotics every day, on time, for months on end. This is a pain in the ass as you can imagine. But if you don't take the meds as scheduled, you're helping the little bugs inside your lungs get use to the antibiotics, and you know the deal about what doesn't kill you only makes you stronger. Yup, having TB sucks in many ways. The resistance problem isn't helped by the people who were only exposed to the disease, but haven't developed it yet. These folks usually take an antibiotic, isoniazid, the same way, for months on end, every day, and these people feel just fine. Not a good recipe for compliance.

Now to understand my plan, just wander into any drugstore on a Friday night. What you'll see before too long will be someone explaining how they lost their pain med....maybe their dog ate it (and somehow had no side effects). They'll be coming in for a refill on a 30 day supply of their Tylenol with Codeine #3 on the 15th day, for the 4th month in a row. They'll be bringing me a 3rd prescription for the same medicine from a 3rd doctor. They'll be explaining how they had to take twice as much because one dose was for their foot pain and the next dose was for their back. Yup....meet the addict. Every drugstore has a few. Gotta be firm with them because they can sense weakness. I've been begged to, propositioned, threatened, offered money on the side, cursed at and more by the addicts. It comes with the territory of having a job that involves working in a room full of narcotics. I'm used to it.

So what's this got to do with me taking a little trip to Norway to get a medal from the king you say? Simple. Three words. Isoniazid with codeine. Can you imagine it? People lining up at the pharmacy on Friday nights, telling me......"you don't understand!!!!!!! I NEED my TB medicine NOW!!!!!!!" The scourge that has been civilization's unwanted companion from time eternal would be banished from our planet within a year, future rap stars hustling isoniazid on the streets, to ensure it will never return. My next plan involves Vicodin and the flu vaccine.

Another Random Day Of Pill Counting Highlights

Karma set her gentle hands upon me and nudged me into consciousness early this day. I knew not why, but I know better than to fight Karma when Karma has plans for you. I pulled back the blinds and was bathed in the brilliant sunshine of a California coastal morning. Perhaps Karma meant to mock me this workday. To force me to look at her brilliance. That didn't seem right though. That's so unlike Karma. I put my fate in her hands and began my day.

I heard it before I even walked through the front door. "WHAT TIME DOES THE PHARMACY OPEN??? I HAVE A TEE TIME!!!!!" It was at that moment I realized why Karma had set me in motion this day earlier than usual. Karma wanted me to go to Starbucks and have a cup of coffee. Bitching about your tee time is probably the best way to ensure that I open right on time when I am running early.

Not that I have anything against golf. It's more the type of assholes who play golf I have something against.

The first prescription of the day was for 36 mg of Concerta, a stimulant used to treat children whose parents suffer from codependency, and 20mg of Ambien, a sleep aid. Right there on the same blank written at the same time by the same doctor. It reminded me of a story I read once about how prison guards would, for their own entertainment, put one inmate from the Crips and one from the Bloods in the yard at the same time knowing they would fight it out gladiator style. I wondered if the doctor just wanted to see which drug would win.

The phone rang and the person said "Oh, I have the wrong number, I wanted to phone in some prescription refills" and hung up. The next caller didn't hang up, and asked me if we carried basketballs. After that though, came the best call of all:

"Oh....is (insert name of other pharmacist) there?"

"No, it's her day off"

"I'll just call back later"

You would have to know this particular customer to know just how sweet those words sounded. She was trained now to want to deal only with the other pharmacist. Finally, I was free of this customer who had been such a bane on my worklife. Free......

Or maybe not. The "clank....clank.....clank..." of the walker making its way up the tile floor announced the entry of another person into my life.

"I'M TIRED OF TRYING TO DEAL WITH THOSE CLOWNS!!! I WANT TO GO TO THE BEST!!!! ARE YOU THE BEST?"

I don't think I lied to him really. I'm definitely the best pharmacy in this mall. Probably the best within a 10 block area or so. He wasn't all that specific, and I'm sure as shit a step up from the store from which he came, which is, in fact, manned by clowns. Sometimes I think the whole reason some drug chains are profitable is because of the humongous tax credits they must receive for hiring the handicapped.

"I LIKE YOU!!!!" Was the last thing walker man said to me before he clanked out the door. I was free for about an hour. Karma giveth and Karma taketh away.

I'm thinking Concerta would shank Ambien and totally make Ambien its bitch.

I Live An Episode Of "The Office"

So, both the district managers came in the store one day. For those of you not in the pharmacy biz I'll tell you management chores in a corpro-pharmacy are usually split into two tracks. A pharmacist DM who is theoretically there to deal with things professional and another DM who is there to deal with everything else. The regular DM usually has some sort of business degree, which means the following story shouldn't surprise you much.

The pharmacy DM comes in and does her thing. Looks through paperwork, does crap on the computer, takes calls from other stores having some sort of crisis, and generally gets in the way of those of us filling prescriptions. They always ask before they leave if there's anything they can do for you, but they never mean it. I decided to test this one.

"Yes" I said. "You can give me a supervisor number." I've said earlier how I've always thought it odd I'm trusted to be alone in a room full of drugs but not to OK a $20 void sale.

I'd been asking for a supervisor number for four years, through three store managers, three district managers, and more pharmacy DM's than I can name. Five minutes later I had one. The fact I was actually able to convince someone in power to make a small, common sense change that would have a big impact on how easy it is to run the pharmacy gave me kind of an endorphin rush. These moments don't happen often. The last time I remember a Pharmacy District Manager doing something helpful was three years and three DM's ago when one of them scored us another refrigerator. I basked in the feeling of a runner's high.

Then the business major came in.

He was still fairly new from his last gig at a retailer that went bankrupt and eager to show he was in charge and ready to bring some of the magic from his last employer to his current one. He whips out some charts or something that purport to show our prescription counts are down and wants some "input from the team as to what might be causing this"

Unfortunately I'm acutely aware I'm the team member who's gotta do the talking. My keystone tech doesn't get paid nearly enough to deal with this crap.

"Well the first thing that comes to mind is the phones" I say. I've written before about my store's phone problems. There had been four day stretches where people were unable to call the store because the guy who fixes things like phone problems didn't work weekends. The best phone function we had for awhile was to periodically go to the back room and reboot the system throughout the work day. Angry customers were telling me they literally spent weeks trying to get through to us.

"That's interesting" says the business major. "Because I do mystery calls to stores to ask how long it would take to have a prescription filled and they tell me not many prescriptions are phoned in"

I swear he said that.

I'm going to set aside the fact that calling a pharmacy to ask how long it will take to fill a prescription is the stupidest goddamn question I can be asked. I can tell you how long it will take if you're here now. I cannot tell you how busy I might be when you decide to come and drop off a prescription at some unknown point in the future.

I'm also going to set aside the utter implausibility that someone would tell this man not many prescriptions are phoned in. Maybe someone did. As some type of joke.

My point here is that I started out this day trying to find a way to diplomatically explain, in a way that wouldn't get me fired, that not having reliable phone service probably has a net negative impact on our business.

I found a way. Because my other choice would have been to suggest the elimination of phones altogether as a cost saving measure that would have minimal impact on sales. That probably would have gotten me promoted, and I don't feel like being on the road all day long.

My Employer Finds A New Way To Crush My Soul, Or I Have Taken The Last Short Step To Becoming Completely Insane. One Of The Two.

The flood that brought back the pain happened about mid-piss, and it had nothing to do with kidney stones. It was a flood of memories, and it was triggered by the fact that the bathroom had finally been cleaned. You see, it would seem my employer has changed the mixture of chemicals they use to sanitize the little boys room, and those that they now use, and I swear I am not making this up, smell a lot like the perfume an ex-girlfriend of mine used to wear.

An ex-girlfriend whose association with me did not end well. At all. Actually it was OK for her, but kinda bad for me. I'm over it now though.

Twitch.....twitch.....why are you looking at me like that? You've never seen a man chug scotch out of a bottle before? Totally over her......shake.....twitch.....

So half my brain was dealing with the memory flood, and the other half was determining it was highly implausible that this woman had ever spritzed a little bathroom cleaner on her pulse points before going out for the evening. This led me to the only logical conclusion possible:

My employer had specifically formulated the scent of its disinfectant to further their goal of breaking me.

The good news is that the infrequency of their bathroom cleaning and the fact I get fewer and fewer chances to take advantage of the facilities amongst the ever increasing crush of pill seeking barbarians will work against their plan. I fully expect in the near future though, they will hire my ex-wife as a pharmacy tech and my alcoholic Dad as perhaps the store manager. My theory is that it saves them money somehow if they can drive me to suicide instead of just firing me or hiring a contract killer.

I only hope the drive will be a short one.

Sometimes When I'm Sad And Blue About Being Single Though, I Sing Myself A Little Song To Cheer Me Up.

It goes a little something like this:

I can do whatever I want
whatever I want
whatever I want

I can do what ever I want
I just left the toilet seat up.

I am master of the remote
I can bang on a pan!
I can fart really loud

Yes yes I can!

'cause I'm single and can do what I want.

A nasty lovers spat
I don't know what that is!
couple politics
that's none of my biz!

yes, that dress
makes you look fat

you know why I can tell you that?

'cause I'm single and can do what I want.

the tempo now dramatically slows, think climax of a Broadway musical number....

Someday I'll die alone......in a pool of my own urine.
But for now its fast cars, freedom and pourin'...............

the scotch
and the gin

every day feels like a big new win........

Because I do

what

ever

I

want.

Actually It's Good I'm Still Single, Because I Have Yet To Have Sex With A Jew

I am a bit of a Michael Moore groupie. After reading this far into the book that shouldn't be a surprise to you. What is surprising to me however is that it took me so long to track down *Blood In The Face,* a documentary Mike did some work on early in his career that features his first cinematic moment of note, an interview with a hot nazi chick "You don't look like a typical Nazi" Mike tells the woman, who is obviously flattered.

At any rate, the film is a look into the world of white supremacist whack jobs. A few minutes in, one of the whack jobs is ranting about Filipinos. This reminded me of the most beautiful woman I ever had the privilege of nailing. That woman's skin felt like velvet and I will never forget it. She was a Filipina, and I still miss her sometimes, even though she was a whack job herself in a different sort of way.

Then one of the Nazi whack jobs starts ranting about mixed-race women. I once was nail-buddies with a woman whose hair would put goosebumps on the skin of any heterosexual male or lesbian. She was absolutely gorgeous and she was half black/half white. Sadly, the nail-buddy experience is now part of my personal history book. Sigh.

The people in the movie spent most of their time ranting about Jews though. Wow they really didn't like Jewish people. Now I have to be honest, I don't think I know any Jewish people in the real world, but I walked away from this film totally convinced that I have to nail one or two. I think to be a complete traitor to my race, I really should complete the trifecta.

Plus I learned from the film that Jews control everything. Which is kinda hot.

I wonder if it would be worth getting circumcised

A Random Day Of Pill Counting Highlights

Why would you ask that? Seriously. If it's 9:00, and you're at the pharmacy, and you see me cranking open the gates, key words......cranking open.......why on Earth would you ask.....

Remember it's 9:00. Pretty much on the button.

......"what time does the pharmacy open?" Shouldn't you be able to at least formulate a pretty good guess based on observational data? And maybe not interrupt me while I'm in the process of opening?

I seriously can't think of a stupider question right now. It's definitely the dumbest one I've been asked in years.

First prescription of the day was for 10 vials of Humalog insulin that had been billed for one. Which means within the first five minutes of business I saved more than an entire days worth of profit. Because I am all about capitalism and profit. How the place functioned before they had the wisdom to hire me I'll never know.

One of the first customers of the day to my trusty technician: "I don't have any prescriptions ready? Good....because I don't need anything, but I thought the computer called me." I seriously think the customer would have bought whatever the computer told them to. The Unabomber tried to tell us this day was coming. Your future enslavement to the machines will be my opportunity for wealth however, because in my never ending pursuit of profit, I think I am going to start a program where I call people in a robotic-sounding voice and order them to come to the store and buy shit.

I think I'll tell them to buy nail clippers. I will not be happy until every person you see on the street is wearing a set of nail clippers around their neck.

A professional dilemma. You overhear a customer ask where the Icy Hot is because he wants to put it on his blood clot. Do you investigate? Find out why he thinks he has a blood clot? Marvel at his ability to walk and talk while some part of his body has evidently been cut off from the vital nourishment that is free flowing blood in its liquid form? Tell him that Icy Hot may be the least effective clot busting drug ever, but the only one covered on the Cigna Health Care formulary?* While I was pondering this the phone rang and I had to take a prescription and my cashier told him Icy Hot was down aisle three. I guess karma really didn't think my involvement was required.

My technician asked me "So what are you doing all weekend?" Offending the three teenage girls at the condom rack who assumed she was talking to them. I'd be offended too. Who says you can't have sex during the week?

Towards the end of the day came the Great Cash Register Summit. The Assistant Manager who's been an Assistant Manager for 10 years came back to take the register till to the office. She couldn't get the drawer to pop open. She tried this. Then that. Then this again. And again. And again. You've heard the old saying about the definition of insanity being doing the same thing over and over again and expecting different results? I always thought that Assistant Manager was bat-shit crazy, and now I had proof. She called the other manager with less than a quarter of her experience to solve the problem. They defined themselves as insane a few more times before they decided to reboot the register. Part of me wanted to help. Kind of. But it was so damn entertaining, and I was kind of offended when they decided to bring the rookie cashier back to ask his insight. It was a full scale summit now. A meeting of the minds. The computers can successfully order us to come in and buy stuff but we are incapable of getting them to open the cash register drawer. The handwriting is on the wall my friends.

The drawer popped open while a woman battling a refill too soon reject had my attention. I will never know all the details of the great cash register summit.

The day ended with a guy popping his head under the gate as I was cranking it shut to ask what time we closed. For some reason that didn't bother me as much.

That was a joke. I'm sure Cigna covers effective clot dissolving medication. I'm also sure that in 2009 they denied coverage for a teenager's liver transplant and then she died. Wait. That wasn't fair. Cigna did change their minds and decide to pay for the transplant. A few hours before she died. Cigna said "This decision was made despite the fact that Cigna had no obligation to do so and despite concluding, based on the information available, that the treatment would be unproven and ineffective and therefore experimental and not covered by the employer's benefit plan,"

Awww.....isn't Cigna sweet? They decided to let a teenage girl try to live even though they had no obligation to do so.

A public health plan would have an obligation to do so. Just sayin'

Worst Sales Rep Ever

So it's an uneventful day in the happy little pill room, and out of the corner of my eye I see what looks like an average numbnut customer fumbling around for an insurance card or something. Wandering over I see instead a lady cleaning up a mess of brochures she dropped on the counter and all over the floor. Turns out she was trying to set up a promotional display for a new sleep aid and was having a little trouble. Never asked if she could set up the display or even bothered to say hello, just came in and started to put stuff on my counter.

Letting the breach of basic etiquette slide, I gathered up a few brochures and asked, "Rozerem, is that the new melatonin agonist I've heard about?"

"Yeah", came the unenthusiastic reply "I really don't see why you just can't take melatonin" Then back to reassembling the display.

It won't surprise anyone in the profession to hear that at that moment the phone rang. When I was done with the call, the super saleslady had moved on, leaving behind a display that was almost put together the way it was designed to be. I wonder where in sales school they teach you that:

1) First impressions aren't that big of a deal

2) The only words you should say are those that talk people out of using the product you are trying to sell.

3) Leaving behind something half-ass is the perfect way to make that shitty first impression have a lasting impact.

The brochure that was to convince people that Rozerem was the answer to their sleep related problems featured a groundhog and what appeared to be Abraham Lincoln on the cover. Seriously. I think when I have a groundhog and Abraham Lincoln coming into my life to explain the importance of a good night's sleep, that pretty much eliminates the need for me to ever try LSD.

Sometimes Big Pharma isn't intimidating at all.

My Fecal Material Is Free.....Free To Soar Amongst The Eagles......

....and Amitiza is the wind beneath its wings. Evidently that is the image that Takeda Pharmaceuticals, the same people that brought you those images of a groundhog playing chess with Abraham Lincoln to plug a sleeping pill, thinks will imbed its drug into the brains of healthcare professionals everywhere. Going through the mailbag the one day I came across a nifty little ad. It featured the word "ACTIVATE" across the top, above a series of green squares, some of which looked like they were starting to be blown upward by the wind.

How could I not be intrigued? I mean, I like to activate stuff just as much as the next guy. The ad was set up in a window-blind kinda way. There was a tab on the right hand side you could pull that slid the window blind thingies over. You then saw the word "RELIEF" next to "ACTIVATE" and the little squares that looked like they were starting to soar upwards turned into little birds rising into the sky.

I now knew that this miracle medicine was the answer to my life's troubles. I wanted....no I NEEDED..... to soar, to break loose of the gridlock of life and rise....rise upwards towards freedom and heaven itself.

I felt in my very soul that Amitiza was for me. Then I saw the ailment Amitiza was meant to treat; chronic idiopathic constipation. The birds were representative of my shit starting to flow.

Even though I have been blessed with regular bowel movements, somehow looking at this ad I still felt the desire to take the drug, and had to read more about it. Maybe in the fine print I would see something about how it enhances the happy feelings scotch gives me. Didn't happen. What I did see was that the most common side effect was nausea, which happened to 31% of people in clinical trials. Actual puking happened in 5%.

So you have a choice between being stopped up and not able to go, and an almost 1 in 3 chance that you'll be trading that for the feeling of having to puke and not being able to. I suppose I can see now why they felt they needed an ad a little "out of the box" for this one. Should my birds ever stop flying though, I think I'll stick with other options.

And Jet Skis Are Free To Ride On My Urine.

That is the type of image the marketing wonks toiling away for Big Pharma thinks will make your doctor prescribe their product. That and shit birds. I swear I'm not lying to you.

First, the required background. If you're a guy, there's a decent chance that if you live to be old, you won't be able to pee as you'd like. As many as 90% of men between 70 and 90 will develop symptoms of Benign Prostatic Hyperplasia, or BPH. Translated to English, that means your prostate gland will swell, constricting the tube that leads from your bladder through your wiener. When this happens, you can't get all the pee out of your bladder, so you feel like you have to go all the time, even though you can't. I'm sure it sucks, but would it really lead you or your doctor to respond to an image of a giant fire hydrant gushing forth, and a jet ski being ridden by a late middle aged couple in the middle of the bountiful liquid coming forth from the fire hydrant? That is exactly the image Sanofi Aventis put forth in an ad to plug its BPH drug Uroxatral.

The fire hydrant was self-evident I suppose, if a bit tasteless, but what on earth was up with the jet ski? Are they trying to say your pee-hole will be so relaxed that you could pass out a watercraft? Who are these people who think it's fun to ride a jet ski in this type of environment? Has the Tidy Bowl Man come out of retirement and decided he likes riding around in the sewage itself, instead of above it like he used to? First we have the chuckle inducing drug name of another med used to treat BPH, Flomax, and now this.

I hope this ad agency never gets the Viagra account

Random Pill Counting Highlights

To Every Thing There Is A Season.......and a time to every purpose under the heaven; A time to be born, and a time to die.

That came from the Bible. I have no problem ripping off God when I need material

My label printer died this day. It wasn't a surprise. We've all saw that it was very sick for quite awhile. It pained me to watch the label printer go through its final phases. Mysterious farting noises, unresponsiveness, chronic misalignment indicative of delusional confusion. It pained me mostly because it meant I had to do three times as much work to get a label on every goddamn vial that was going out the door. My label printer's pain is over now, the heroic efforts of my employer's electronic maintenance department to save the $60 or so it probably would have cost them to replace it came to naught. The carcass of my label printer was carried out this afternoon.

Fucking piece of shit.

If only the printer would have had the robust health of the store's public address system. Not a damn thing wrong with that piece of equipment. And it's not the least bit shy either, never hesitating to announce something like "I NEED A PRICECHECK ON HEINZ KETCHUP 32 OUNCE TWINPACK!!!!!" every other time I am talking to a person about their prescription or trying to decode a doctor's message on the voicemail. Today the overbearing obnoxiousness of the PA system had the added bonus of seemingly being manned by a drunk woman. Seriously. I know drunkenness like few other subjects my friends and the lady up front totally gave the impression of having hit up the sauce. I summoned one of the high-school age clerks pretending to stock the shelves.

"Hey.....hey B, go smell N"

"What?"

"Seriously. She sounds totally drunk. See if you can smell it on her breath. Ask if you can borrow a pen or something."

This is why it's great to be at a level above that of regular worker, but not quite that of management expected to run things. Because I can send people up to sniff the front end checker not out of any concern for the well being of the store, but solely for self-amusement purposes.

The sniff test came back negative. I am still working on alternate explanations.

I do do professional stuff though. Like help the man who told me he got an antibiotic the other day and was sure "it has just decimated my system." He then asked if I knew anything about amoxicillin. I explained to him amoxicillin does tend to come up in our profession's schooling and then listened for a good 3 or 4 minutes how he had "this thing that's up in my sinuses, and down in my throat and you know.....cough cough. The cough was faked for my benefit. The monologue ended with. "I've been getting better the last three days"

Just to help my colleagues out there reading this. Forget the definition of "decimated" you may have learned in high school. It now means "isn't curing me quite as fast as I'd like to be cured"

My technician asked for help reading the directions on a prescription she was typing.

"Prior to semen collection" I told her. She then washed her hands.

The day ended with another reminder of the fragility of life. My pen died a natural death. This was a surprise. Pens in my world as a rule have short, violent existences. They are chewed on from the moment they enter my hands. Their points are slammed against prescription pads when nurses make my life far harder than it should be and they were at one time quite often thrown across the room. Nowadays they are usually thrown straight into the floor so fewer people see. The Azor pen made it all the way to the end of its ink cartridge today though. It was a tough bastard, and it will be missed.

Not as much as if I hadn't scored a new Viagra pen though. Karma saw fit to provide me with a new Viagra pen and that means this goes down in the books as a good day.

The Viagra pen won't be chewed on though, as I can't seem to put the Viagra pen in my mouth. Not that there would be anything wrong with that.

A Twofer Of Random Pill Counting Highlights

I tried to blow my nose and immediately clogged up my ears. This has happened from to time to time before, for like a second or two, but this time the clog wasn't going anywhere. I tried a big yawn, I stuck my pinky in and wiggled it around, I popped in some gum that I realized too late was an....what is the word.....rather....exotic....flavor one of my technicians had brought over from India, but it was all as effective at clearing out my ear as the Airborne is at preventing colds. I started to wonder if maybe a piece of snot had gotten blown up next to my eardrum. Customers do not wait for you to resolve your personal problems however, and there was a man forging his way to the pharmacy to demand my attention.

He asked me about earwax removable drops. I swear. When I asked him to repeat what he was saying I think he might have thought I was making fun of him, but I honestly could not have been more empathetic at the moment. I was starting to resign myself to a life of silence.

Until the PA went off. Losing half your hearing brings the store's PA system to almost a bearable level. Bearable in volume. Not necessarily in content. The announcement went something like this:

"Ummmm.....yeah......for the owner of a large dog who asked someone to watch him, it's now run over to Petco....the large dog......that.....a customer wanted watched.......ummmm.....it's now.....over at.....um.......Petco. The large dog. Thank you."

It was the cashier whom I was convinced was drunk yesterday. I sent a clerk back to sniff her again.

My deafness and the saga of the large dog were not the biggest news of this day however. That distinction belongs to a development in my employer's prescription transfer gift card program. For what seemed like an eternity, my employer offered a $25 gift card to customers who transfer their prescriptions from another pharmacy. And when they say "customers who transfer a prescription from another pharmacy" what they of course meant was "any customer who asks for one." Transfers, new prescriptions, refills, buying something the syndicated health columnist in the local newspaper recommended, the tone set from our higher ups has been clear. Give 'em a card and shut them up. Today we may have finally found the limit to my employer's generosity though.

A woman demanded a gift card for transferring her two prescriptions to another store. Let me repeat that. Someone wanted us to pay her for taking her prescriptions and having them filled somewhere else. She didn't get a card, and this one might stick.

Might I said.

My ear unclogged and I wasn't sure if it was my imagination that made me feel a chunk of something go down my throat I was forced to swallow. I vowed to only breathe through my mouth from now on like the stupid people do. I walked over to the in window to wait on the nervous looking man, who presented me with a prescription made out for Keflex and Vicodin.

"Can you just enter the antibiotic?" He asked. Huh. Sometimes water does go uphill I guess.

"Sure, I'll just put the other one on hold in your profile for you, if you decide you want it just let us know."

"No!!!"

He explained that he was a recovering addict, that he had told the people at the emergency room this when he was admitted, and that when he saw the Vicodin on his prescription he asked the nurse to scratch it off. Whereupon the nurse told him just not to fill it. I wondered if my local hospital had a program where they might stuff t-bone steaks into the discharge packages of vegans and told the man that the Vicodin order no longer existed.

So the day ended with a customer begging not to get Vicodin. Talk about a disturbance in the force. I had high hopes for tomorrow. High hopes. Ha. I just got that. I kill me.

Real Words Spoken By A Real Customer.

UMMM......YEAH.......I TAKE ADDERALL........AND.......UH.......KLONOPIN.......AND......VICODIN..... TAKE THE VICODIN BECAUSE IT HELPS ME CONCENTRATE.......AND THIS HERE'S A PRESCRIPTION FOR PROZAC. MY DOCTOR SAID IT WOULD HELP GROW BRAIN CELLS. IS THAT RIGHT?????

Oh severely misguided customer, you have no idea how sincerely... how deeply....how with every last bit of a bit of my very soul I wish that Prozac grew brain cells. I would give it away for free. I would put it in the water. I would bake it in bread. I would saturate the atmosphere with nebulized Prozac if only it were so. My dear sir, you and I, we're not so different, we both long for something........anything, that will allow your brain to grow out of it's current sorry state. What a wonderful dream to have.....

Until that day comes though my good man, might I suggest you at least stop killing the brain cells you do have. I swear I could pick out the particular brand of gin that was lending it's aroma to your breath. I'm not sure if that says more about your love of alcohol or mine.

A Little Secret Of The Profession. The FDA Doesn't Always Make A Company Prove Their Medicine Is Effective Against Disease.

Some of you reading this will now think I'm out of my mind. That proof of effectiveness is the cornerstone of the entire drug-approval process, and you would be right, to a point. The FDA does indeed require evidence of effectiveness for a new drug to be approved, but there are times when it requires zero proof of effectiveness against an actual disease.

Meet our friend Mr. Surrogate Marker. He makes this possible. I think the best illustration of Mr. Surrogate Marker and how he can lead you off the path of the scientific method can be done with the help of a little time travel. So climb with me into the wayback machine to 16th century London, ground zero for culture and cutting edge medicine of the time:

The scene, The Academy of Smart Fellow Medicine, London's finest hospital:

Doctor wearing a wig: Zodooks and other curses! Another case of ill humored corpsucular spirits! It has been the leading cause of death in our fair city for a score of year now! Assistant! Knock that rat off the table and prepare the leeches to suck a pint of blood from the patient immediately!

A scantily clad wench enters through the office door, carrying an armful of boxed lunches:

My good doctor! I bring you tidings and wonderful news! A breakthrough in the treatment of ill humored corpsucular sririts (IHCS) from my superiors at the general meydicyne and surgical company!

Doctor Wig (staring at the wenches breasts): Tell me more of this breakthrough young lass!

Wench: We call it Warfarene. And it decreases the amount of time needed to bleed a pint of blood from an IHCS patient by over 50%! Here are many studies to prove this from the Royal Leeching Society. And many quill feathers you may use as pens.

Doctor Wig: Huzzah! Everyone knows decreasing the amount of time necessary to bleed a pint of blood helps in the treatment of IHCS!

Wench: It is a glorious day! Soon the future of IHCS patients will be long and prosperous!

As you can probably guess. The future of IHCS patients was in fact short and wracked with misery. That is because the good Dr. Wig fell into the trap of the surrogate marker. Surrogate markers are easy to identify. If you can fill in x and y in the following sentence:

"Everyone knows x helps in the treatment of y"

You've got yourself a surrogate marker. Let's try a few:

"Everyone knows lowering LDL cholesterol helps in the treatment of heart disease"

Vytorin and Zetia are two medicines that undeniably have been proven to lower LDL cholesterol. Eight years after they came to market however, there is no proof that either lowers the risk of heart attack or helps heart patients live longer. In January of 2008, a study designed to show the drugs shrink arterial plaque was declared a failure.

"Everyone knows lowering a patient's blood sugar helps in the treatment of diabetes"

Avandia unquestionably lowers a diabetic's blood sugar. It also increases the risk for a heart attack. If your diabetes improves and your heart explodes, you're just as dead.

Surrogate markers aren't always bad. When other evidence is thin and not many options are on the table, knowing that a med has been proven to shrink your tumor (but not necessary lengthen your life) is a way better option than a bottle of shark cartilage. For diseases such as hypertension, high cholesterol, and diabetes though, where there are many proven disease-modifying treatments already available, approval based solely on surrogate marker evidence makes no sense. Let's see what happened when the FDA grew a pair and stood up to Big Pharma's surrogate marker play:

"Everyone knows raising HDL cholesterol helps in the treatment of heart disease, and our drug raises HDL, so it must be very helpful" said Pfizer.

"Prove it" said the FDA.

So Pfizer reluctantly did a large scale study measuring actual outcomes in actual patients, and found that its drug, torcetrapib, which did indeed raise HDL, also increased the risk of death by 60% Remember that the next time someone tells you about the evils of government regulation and the virtues of the free market.

Be careful out there friends. Don't stop taking anything without talking to your doctor first, but remember your interest is in maintaining your health, while a drug company's interest is in accumulating each and every last dollar it can. Sometimes your interest will match the drug company's, but other times it will not.

Be careful.

After Reading That Last Chapter, You May Start To Think I Spend My Workdays Reading And Analyzing Scientific Work. Let Me Clear That Up With A Reminder Of What A Typical Workday Is Like.

Power surge. It sounds like a good thing. Like maybe I turned up some sort of personal booster knob that allows me to fill prescriptions just a little bit faster, but no, a power surge is a very bad thing. A power surge can fry your fax machine, which is what we found out at my workplace. It can also knock out the electricity in the part of town where the nearest store in your giant corporate pharmacy chain is located, which happened as well. This means all the familiar lunatics I deal with were joined by a pack of unfamiliar pill craving lunatics from the other side of town. It was like a lunatic regional meeting.

At about the midpoint of the agenda, I get a phone call. A woman evidently upset that she couldn't attend the meeting in person, but determined to take part in the festivities. "YOUR CARTS ARE ALL OVER THE STREET!!!!"

For a person to get me on the phone, they have to navigate an incredibly complex voice mail system that makes it clear at several points they will be talking to the pharmacy, and giving them the option, again at more than one point, of veering off this path and talking to someone in the general store.

"Are they blocking traffic?"

"NO! THEY ARE ALL OVER THE SIDEWALK!"

Knowing that our store was physically a long way from a sidewalk, and that any stray carts from our place almost certainly would become the property of the local homeless population before they got anywhere near a sidewalk, and that the now powerless store, five miles away mind you, was right next to the street, I ask the nice lady, "ma'am are you talking about the store at address X? You're talking to the store at address Y"

"I DON'T CARE! I'M CALLING THE POLICE!"

This was supposed to frighten me. I thought about why. Were the police going to come and arrest the shopping carts? Would they be booked and thrown in a cell without access to counsel? Might giant corpo-pharmacy's shopping carts end up as bitches to the Crips, traded to the Bloods for a carton of cigarettes?

I never got a call from the carts asking for bail money. As a matter of fact, I never heard of the carts again. I fear they may have been stripped of their habeas corpus rights. I hope they don't end up in Guantanamo.

We live in dark times.

The Impending Arrest Of My Shopping Carts Made Me Seriously Think About Another Career. I Was Surprised At How Simple The Solution Seemed.

I decided I should become a professional gold miner. Seriously. I live in California you see, and there's no way they've gone over every inch of California since the original gold rush. Back in 1849 people were shorter, they didn't have access to the variety of foods to provide vitamins and energy that we have today, and they didn't have cell phones. Think how much more efficient a modern gold miner could be! I'm sure there still has to be a big chunk of gold out there somewhere, but I'm not greedy. At current prices I would only need to find like 5 ounces a month to have enough money to get by. How the hell hard could that be? Five ounces!

The hours would also be very agreeable. Basically, anytime there's daylight. Once I find my first ounce, I'll buy one of those little headlamp thingies and have 24/7 capability. I suppose I'll need one of those pans or something too.

And if worse comes to worse, and all I find is fools gold, then I'll just find some fool to sell it to. One thing my pharmacy career has taught me is that there is no shortage of fools. I'm gonna head to the Sierra Foothills as soon as I sober up. I'll try not to laugh at you suckers when I'm rich.

UPDATE- I originally wrote that around midnight. It is now approximately 3:15 AM and so far I have checked both under my bed and in the hall closet, and I have found no gold. It may be because I do not yet have one of those pans. Should these disappointing results continue, I may be forced to expand my search to silver, or perhaps uranium if I can get a good market price.

I Woke Up The Next Afternoon And Realized I Was No Gold Miner, But Still Wanted To Be Rich. I Decide To Take A Different Course.

Not many can pull off up and starting a brand new career by the time gray starts to settle in around the temples. Even if those temples are covered in thick, fabulous, non-bald hair, and not even if I am one of the hottest 40ish men on the planet. No my friends, around my age, people start to get defined for what they've been, not what they will be. So it may well be time to accept that my career path is set, to stop wasting my time on cockamamie dreams of being the next Carl Bernstein, and to spend it instead concentrating on becoming the best pharmacist I can be.

Which leads me to two words: Elvis Pharmacy. Who the hell wouldn't want their prescription filled by Elvis?

You need a niche to succeed in today's marketplace, and while Elvis has been done every which way since he took his terminal poop, having him behind the pharmacy counter would be a first for both The King of Rock and Roll and the drugstore business. Not to mention the professional dignity of a pharmacist wearing a sequined jumpsuit and sunglasses is a good two or three steps up from the quickie drive throughs, the Maalox name tags, and the "Your prescription ready in 20 minutes!" barking over the store's PA offered by today's pimps of the profession. And really, who better to counsel you on that Percocet prescription?

"Now you listen to the king" I'll say while looking over the top of my rose-tinted eyewear. "You only take these if you're really hurtin.' The king didn't do that, the king took them whenever he wanted to, and look how the king turned out. "

My God this idea has "license to print money" written all over it. The Elvis demographic isn't getting any younger, and if old people buy anything, it's pills and muscle rubs. Elvis would charge extra to apply the muscle rub. Of course The Elvis Pharmacy would be in Las Vegas, and any town where you can pick up your dry cleaning at two in the morning is a natural fit for myself, who is writing these words at that very hour.

I could also easily gain 40 to 50 pounds and still play the role. Plus I would get to wear a cape. It would involve a lot of prescription transfers, as it would be the tourists who would mainly be begging me to sell them shit, but this could be dealt with; even become part of the Elvis Pharmacy experience. Listen in as Elvis calls your square drugstore back home.

Those of you in the profession, you have been warned. Don't be surprised to get a call from Elvis.

After Another Drinking Binge, I Have Second Thoughts About The Elvis Pharmacy.

Copyright and trademark issues are sure to be a problem, and frankly, I think it would require a lot of movement on my part. I'm not a big fan of movement right now. I just spent the last 5 minutes staring at a bug climbing up the wall. I'm sure that's not a good sign. I have a new idea for the pharmacy of the future:

You walk through the door and into the darkness. A spring on the door ensures that it shuts quickly behind you, minimizing your exposure to any light other than the solitary candle I have lit on the counter. I am dressed in black. The walls are black. You are my regular customer only because the big chain up the street takes an hour to fill your prescription and all you care about is getting it in 5 minutes. You lay the order on the counter.

"Levaquin" I say in a tone distracted and distant. "Of course I will help you, but of course you know the Levaquin will only delay the inevitable. Life itself is a futile event my friend. Yet we struggle on"

As I turn away to fill your prescription you notice the one picture on the wall. It is of Homer Plessy.

Miles Davis' "Kind Of Blue" forms an oddly synergistic auditory compliment to the sound of your prescription label being printed. I seemly emerge out of nowhere to tell you your cure is ready. You ask only why your co-pay is so high.

"Why is anything?" I say. "Why is anything............" my voice tails off as the cash register spits out your credit card approval.

"Enjoy your gift." I say softly as you make your way to the door. As the light of day blinds you while you step back onto the street you think you hear me say......

"Enjoy your struggle. It's the only one you'll get"

Yeah. I'll be totally rich with this idea. Beats the crap out of all the happy pie in the sky bullshit every other drugstore is shining up your ass.

If nothing else my drugstore of darkness will leave me far more emotionally satisfied. I'm going to stare at the wall now for awhile.

I Sober Up For A Couple Days, Don't Like It, And Decide Maybe I Should Just Hope For The End.

So 48 hours without alcohol was enough really. Ending a late night at work and not having to go back until mid-afternoon the next day I really didn't see the point in not starting the scotch a-flowin'. So I popped the cork on a bottle of Laphroaig and put on my favorite Jimi Hendrix vinyl, a live recording from the Isle of Wight festival in 1970. Because of organizational fuckups that day, Jimi didn't take the stage until almost 3 in the morning, and the record has a total 3 in the morning feel about it, which was perfect, because that was the approximate time my one-man party got started. Three LP's later, I accidentally opened the curtains and saw a blanket of the most brilliant blood red clouds covering the eastern sky I could imagine. Red sky in morning sailors warning you know, and these clouds were far beyond red. I almost wish I had paid the extra money to have this book printed in color now so you could look for yourself, but I'm a tightass, so if you want to see you'll have to drop me an email and ask for the picture. My jaw dropped in amazement and I came to the only logical conclusion a scotch-fuzzed brain jam packed full of Jimi could.

The gates of hell were opening. This was the end of the world. I was free at last.

O reader, can you even comprehend the complete and total body orgasm this thought sent through me? I mean, not only was the world finally about to know if this was the first or second coming, but I wouldn't have to be at work tomorrow! Who could possibly need a prescription on the day of the Apocalypse? I was about to trade the torments of my customers for the plagues of hell. In the words of George Jefferson, I was moving on up baby!

Then the clouds parted, I passed out, and the alarm went off a few hours later. I went to work as usual.

-A man tried to use his third $25 prescription transfer coupon and argued over the meaning of "limit one per person" for half an hour.

-I was asked 15 times in 45 minutes where the bathroom was.

-An old woman called to say she didn't have her medicine. While she acknowledged that she must have bought it once I told her we had her signature on file as having picked it up less that a week ago, the problem I was supposed to solve was I'M SICK AND I DON'T FEEL LIKE GOING OUT TO THE CAR AND LOOKING FOR IT!

-On the bright side, an Asian dude honest to God bowed to me after asking me something or other about his Flexeril. Maybe things will turn around.

Or maybe the world will end tonight.

A guy's gotta have dreams.

Random Pillcounting Highlights

So I wasn't sure what to do with this guy. Last time he was in the store he told me all about how he was starting a company where he "would be hiring all sorts of pharmacists and techs" and offered me a job. That wasn't the problem, although I did just condense into one sentence what took him a good twenty minutes to say.

The time before that he told me how he was going off to Bermuda for a modeling job. The time before that how creepy it was to wake up in a mental hospital "full of the really crazy people." You have an idea of the problem now. He was a regular customer, and I had no idea how one would distinguish him from the really crazy people.

Except this time he was asking me about peanut allergies. He told me he was deathly allergic to peanuts and he had just eaten a peanut butter sandwich. He asked me what he should do.

"Well if you're as allergic as you say you are you're gonna have to go to the ER" I said. It was the correct answer. "Deathly allergic" he did say. And even though I knew damn well he wasn't, it was the answer to his question.

Holy shit the look on his face was priceless. And the way he sprinted out of the store. Who knew anaphylaxis was the key to a personal best time in the 100 meters.

Lesson to you dear customer. I am only as good as the questions I am asked.

About an hour later I hear, "So what is this medicine for?"

Sweet. If I am only as good as the questions I am asked, It was now time for me to shine baby.

"To treat high cholesterol" Hell yeah. Mr. Pharmacist. Answering pharmacist questions. Hear me roar.

"Why would my doctor give me a medicine for high cholesterol?" My roaring stopped and I went right back into "what do I do with this guy?" mode. I didn't want to be a smart ass. Honest I didn't, but I am only as good as the questions I am asked.

"Because he thinks your cholesterol is too high"

My reward was a stone-faced death glare. Who knew elevated cholesterol was the key to total muscle and cerebral paralysis.

Headed into the homestretch of the workday now I was:

"Can I get a refill?"

"Sure, what's your name?"

"Oops, oh no"

Guy's Mom hated him I guess. Or named him after what was said after the condom broke.

"I have a question" Time to get it up again.

"It says here to take four times a day, but it would be more natural for me to take it three, so that's what I should do, right?"

They say everything is negotiable, including now, evidently, the half life of Penicillin.

But not my quitting time. That is never negotiable. I slammed the gate down after that one, woofed down a sub to keep from starving to death, and made a beeline home to commemorate this day with a tumbler of scotch.

And a peanut. This day definitely deserves to be remembered with a peanut.

A Customer Cracks The Secret Code Needed To Obtain Coverage In The American Health Care System.

One of the great joys of my profession is the fact that while other healthcare professionals may have a little sign in front of the receptionist saying that payment is expected at the time services are rendered, few have the ability to file and adjudicate your health insurance claim on the spot, instantly determining your eligibility and financial liability. Customers appreciate this, and it never fails to lead to many a lively discussion during the workday regarding the scope and amount of their coverage.

What I just said in that last sentence is that customers bitch about their insurance coverage. A lot. Many times at high volume.

The conversations are usually very predictable, and over the general din of pharmacy sounds this afternoon I hear one going on in the background. It's kind of like the pharmacy equivalent to crickets chirping outside a country cabin late in a summer's evening, just part of the expected background noise:

"Sir your insurance company says your coverage has expired."

"WHAT?!!"

"Blue Cross says you're no longer covered. Do you have a new card?"

"No" The customer usually then will just stand there, expecting that that answer will still get them their meds at their usual co-pay. It must be explained again to them at this point that without a valid insurance card, they are liable for the entire cost of their prescription.

This is what the customer said next, complete and unedited. I double checked with my keytstone tech to make sure I heard him correctly:

"There was a senior citizen behind me last time, would that have made any difference?"

I had no choice. I instantly stepped in and reinstated the man's insurance coverage. He had a senior citizen behind him last time. He had figured out the Da Vinci code of health care. What every insurance company employee and health care professional knows and is sworn never to tell. Senior Citizen behind you = full coverage. Having an old geezer stand behind every American was actually the cornerstone of presidential candidate John McCain's health care plan. He knew the secret you see, being an old geezer himself.

I still don't know exactly what point the customer was trying to make, and I hadn't had any scotch in a week.

The streak ended that night.

I've Been Thinking A Lot About How Good A Lighthouse Operator I Would Be, And I Don't Know Why.

I don't mean I don't know why I would be a good lighthouse operator. There is no doubt in my mind I would be the most kick-ass lighthouse operator in maritime navigation history. I could sit there, at the top of my lighthouse all day long, with a book or something, and when I saw a ship on the horizon, I would know in the marrow of my bones that there would be no way it would hit any rocks. Because I would have a backup light bulb next to me. Just in case.

It wouldn't be all business though. As the ships passed by I could tap out things like "You suck" in Morse code using my giant light. If the ship's Captain figured it out, he wouldn't be mad, because I had done such a good job of making sure he didn't become grounded, and because he would realize that injecting a little fun into the day is one of the things that made me the world's best lighthouse operator.

They'd probably put me in the goddamn lighthouse operator Hall of Fame.

What I mean is that I don't know exactly why these thoughts became so embedded in my mind all the sudden. I've known for years what a good lighthouse operator I would be, but for some reason now, I can't get the thought out of my mind. Maybe the lighthouse is actually some sort of phallic symbol, and I realized today that the way to safe harbor for someone I know is through my penis. I think I should use one of those glow in the dark condoms if that turns out to be the case.

Highlights From A Random Day's Pill Counting Action

The day started with an eerie silence. Ominous. Not to mention no messages on the voicemail. There are never no messages on the voicemail. The silence continued and 15 minutes into it I knew something was dreadfully wrong.

The phones were dead again. So dead their corpse was cold. And while it was nice to be able to start the day being able to keep up with the workload those at the home office say we should be able to handle for a change, I knew that disaster was looming.

I will pause here and point out that I noticed the impeding disaster 15 minutes into my shift, and that the store opens an hour before the pharmacy. The numbnuts up front had not taken a phone call in an hour and 15 minutes and didn't have the slightest idea anything was wrong. Probably because they never took the class I did my third year in college entitled "How to tell if the phone is ringing."

I stepped into the leadership void and emailed the corpro-help desk. Disaster was avoided. I stared the day by saving the store.

The first phone call of the day was from a dentist who wanted to phone in a prescription for diazepam, 20mg an hour before the customer's dental appointment. A whopper of a dose. The customer was already taking temazepam 60mg at bedtime. A whopper of a dose. I told the dentist this and the dentist had no idea what the problem could be.

Let's pause again and have everyone not in the profession play a game. I'll call it "See if you're smarter than a dentist" Here are the rules; look at the last three letters in the name of the two meds the customer above would be taking and see if you have any idea what the problem could possibly be. If so, you're smarter than a dentist.

So I started the day by saving the store and then by saving a customer. That's what I do. I save stuff. Which is why I make so goddamn much.

Overheard as the day's routine prescription filling got under way:

Customer: "Where is the corn medicine?"

Front-end clerk: "I think over by the seeds"

I now have some sympathy for the customers who insist on asking only me where the random shit they want to buy is located.

"Oh I'm in a lot of pain!!" said the customer who came in shortly before lunchtime. "Where are your stomach medicines!!??"

"Down aisle 2" Replied my keystone tech.

"What do you recommend!!!???"

"Let me have you talk to the pharmacist"

"I don't have time!!! I'm in too much pain!!!"

The extra time involved, I will point out, would be about how long it would take for the customer and/or myself to bridge the approximately 5 yards between me and my keystone tech. I always wondered why insurance company helpdesks felt the need to tell people if they were calling due to an emergency to hang up and dial 911. As I watched the stomach lady run out of the store empty-handed, I understood.

About an hour later someone called and asked what "buy one, get one free" meant, which made me really happy I made the effort to fix the phones.

In the background Barry Manilow sang "Daybreak," and I could not help but to hum along. Someday I will tell you the story of how Barry Manilow put a scar on my soul perhaps deeper than the one left by the little plastic stunt motorcycle.

Tied up on the phone again, I heard a customer ask if he should take his naproxen with food. I banged on the counter to get my tech's attention and nodded "yes." If you're a pharmacy student, take heed. Your professors won't tell you this, but some days, that's as close as you're gonna get to having an opportunity to counsel someone in the real world.

The day ended with a 5-minute till closing time phone call.

"Do you sell something to measure the downward pressure being put on a jar, like peanut butter, when you open it?"

I cannot convey to you with words the urgency that was in this person's voice.

"No ma'am, I'm sorry, we don't"

"I guess I should ask a physics teacher, huh?"

I started the day by saving the phones, which I thought was a good idea at the time.

Highlights From A Second Random Day Of Pill Counting

The day always starts with the checking of the voicemail. First message of the day; "Um.....hello?.......hello?....." The voice was soft and pleading, seeking help, or maybe just human companionship, at 2:34 in the morning, which was when the time stamp told me this person had connected with the machine. "Hello?....." A little softer this time. The person was giving up. Then a little click. The machine had won.

The next voicemail, in its entirety; "What kind of message should I leave?" Well my dear customer, the answer to that question is really constrained only by the limits of your imagination. The day's weather forecast might be nice, or maybe some news headlines, just in case I woke up late and missed this information on my way into the store. Or maybe you could go a little avant-garde, that would be cool. I once had someone play Spinal Tap's "Sex Farm" into the voicemail machine. So far I think that's been the coolest voicemail I've ever received, but I'm sure with a little inspiration dear customer, you can top it.

11 hours and 50 minutes to go.

First customer of the day had an urgent complaint. The kind that had to go to a person of authority. Since I'm basically Sulu sitting in the captain's chair when Kirk, Spock, and the guy you've never seen before who will be shortly killed are away from *The Enterprise*, the task fell to me:

"My wife's been getting loads of free stuff here, cartloads, and I need it to stop. We've been divorced 42 years and I'm tired of her using my good name."

Once again I could almost identify the brand of gin on his breath. At first I thought Bombay Sapphire, but that was probably just because I wanted some Bombay Sapphire so badly at the moment. After more objective sniffing, I was sure it was the cheap Seagram's.

"I'll take care of it." I assured the man I was insanely jealous of for being able to get away with being drunk at 9:30 in the morning. And that was that. Being Sulu isn't so hard sometimes.

11 hours 30 minutes to go.

A customer spent a good 5 minutes trying to convince me the house brand Tylenol PM and brand-name Excedrin were the same thing. He was arguing like his life depended on it. I wondered why he was so desperate, and I actually kept the conversation going longer than I normally would have just to see if I could find some reason why this was such a vital issue to him. I never did, so I finally ended it with a "well they are both pain relievers, but this one will make you drowsy."

That got me a death glare from the desperate customer. He had failed in his mission to bring me over to his point of view.

Customer call: "Yeah.....I need my Septra refilled.....I'll spell it for you...... o-m-e-p-r-a-z-o-l-e."

For those of you not in the profession, Septra is an antibiotic. Omeprazole is used to treat acid reflux in the stomach.

Doctor call: Yeah I'm phoning in a new prescription.....blah blah blah.......

Me: OK, just this time or do you want additional refills?

"Additional refills" Then a dead silence. I let the silence go on for awhile to see if it would sink in.

"Any particular number of additional refills?"

I'd never had a doctor call me an asshole before. I was feeling a little unprofessional about my snarkiness until he did that.

Doctor call Number 2: "Yeah.....um.....Mr. Smith needs a refill of his Lipitor and the doctor OK'd it. Can you get that faxed over?"

Me: "You just said he OK'd it"

Nurse Dumbass: "So you'll send the fax?"

Me: "Uh, no, you just told me he OK'd it. How many times?"

Nurse Dumbass: "What?"

Me: And what was your name?

"Nurse Dumbass"

It went in as OK'd per Nurse Dumbass 1 time. No fax was ever sent.

6 hours to go.

A person called 3 times within 15 minutes to see if we had 180 tablets of Oxycontin 10 milligram. "The orange ones" It was very important they be orange. When you start getting calls like that on a Friday my friends, you don't need access to a window; you know the sun has just gone down.

Dusk was confirmed by the next call. "Yeah, I want some Viagra, but I don't have a prescription. What should I do?"

Let the Friday night begin.

A customer asked me if the KY jelly could be found with the shaving cream. I so wanted to know what connection was being made in the customers mind between KY jelly and shaving cream, but I was interrupted by someone who asked where the diabetic candy was.

I hate diabetics. The fact you think you're entitled to candy no matter your health condition is a big reason why you're in the position you're in fatass. Now I'll never know the mystery of the KY jelly shaving cream. Thanks for that.

My last customer was in a jam. He had left his Lexapro on the other side of the country and wanted to know if I might be able to fill it here. Easy

184

enough when you work for a big-ass chain with a shared database. The customer was very grateful for this. "My wife was ready to overnight them to me" he said as I rang out his purchase. Meaning his wife was on the other side of the country. The man then also refilled his Cialis, which you can think of as a long-acting version of Viagra, and bought some condoms.

So ended the Friday. For me. Although I'm sure the festivities continued all around town as I slept.

What The Heck, Let's Make It A Pill Counting Highlight Trilogy

Like I've said, the day always starts with the checking of voice mails left from the previous night. There were six on the machine. Five of them were from one of my neighbors. This neighbor can look out of her front window and see my car in the parking lot. All five of the messages wanted to know if we were open yet. Because it's way easier evidently to navigate my employer's voicemail labyrinth than it is to look out of your window to see if I've left for work yet.

If anyone out there knows a good Realtor, please drop me a line.

The sixth voice mail message was, in it's entirety, "I just need my Premarin filled, that's the only message I have" That was every bit of information someone out there thought I needed to fill their prescription. So I just filled some random person's Premarin and declared mission accomplished.

The first written prescription of the day was for Tobradex, which Tricare, the entity responsible for protecting the health of those we've hired to snuff out the health of others, seemed to believe was available in a generic form. It would be shortly, but currently it was not. I took something positive away from the experience though, learning that navigating the Tricare, ahem, "help" desk is a good way to kill an hour. Whenever I'm bored and need to kill some time and find myself without access to a crossword puzzle or something, I'll just call the Tricare helpdesk from now on.

First numbnut question of the day came during the hour I was doing battle with the entity that covers the people who do battle; "WHERE ARE THE COTTON BALLS????" screamed in the ear that wasn't on hold.

"Aisle two, under the sign that says cotton balls"

The customer then thanked me for insulting them. Be very careful about pulling this maneuver my friends, and don't ever do it unless you have the security of a pharmacist license.

The community college dropout who runs the cash office gave us a register drawer with no nickels, thereby providing a clue as to why he didn't make the community college cut. "We need change in the pharmacy" called my trusty technician.

Someone tried to phone in a fake prescription for Vicodin with instructions of "must last one month" I thought that was a nice touch.

Actual question from an actual customer: "Yeah, on this painkiller here, it says to take 1 or 2 every 6 hours, how will I know when I should take 2?"

Think that was the dumbest question I had all day? Not even close. Here's the days winner:

"This label says to take 1 tablet. How do I take 1 tablet?"

I shit you not. I spent a good week memorizing the Krebs cycle some time in 1990 so I could be prepared to tell someone how to take a tablet.

"We need change in the pharmacy" called out my technician.

I was once again given a demonstration that my lingual skills are not nearly cunning enough as the old Hispanic man showed me a box of Monistat and asked "Will she still be a lady?"

I really didn't think the old man thought the Monistat was some sort of over the counter sex change device, but I was without a clue as to what he was trying to ask, until my trusty technician stepped in. "He wants to know if she'll still be a virgin" she said. I should have known, as the word "Monistat" does translate loosely into Spanish as "filthy cum-drenched whore"

Customer to me: "Do you have a fever? You look like you have a fever." They then moved on down the aisle, never giving me a chance to tell them if I had a fever or not.

My trusty technician once again called for change in the pharmacy, but change did not come, the only result of her pleas were that they brought nickels and ones and pennies, but not once did they bring any fundamental change, so it looks like I am destined for more of the same tomorrow.

Stick with the Gyne-Lotrimin if you want to maintain your virginity.

You May Have Realized By Now I Do Not Intend For This Book To Be A Vehicle Of Non-Partisanship. There Was A Time Though, When I Was A Republican.

Seriously. It all started with a hate mail. A hate mail I should have expected. I freely use the word "liberal" you see, and using the word "liberal" in turn of the 21st century America is like waving a red flag in front of a bull. Except in this case the bull is usually a balding, middle aged, paunchy know it all white guy. Think of the guy who doesn't bat an eye when you tell him his Viagra isn't covered on his insurance plan then whips out his credit card. That kind of guy. I used the "L" word once in some of my writing, so sure enough right on cue the next morning this was waiting in my mailbox:

> How can you call yourself a liberal? Your (sic) a Pharmacist, in the top 10% of all incomes in the good 'ole US of A. Do you like being taxed to death to fund all the sick lame and lazy people in this country. That is what your average tax and spend liberal wants. I hope you feel good about being a "liberal" every time a worthless state mediciad recipient comes into your Pharmacy. At least you will know where that 35% of your patcheck (sic) is going. If the liberals have there way it will be closed (sic) to 60%. At least then Mary Rottencrotch and her 16 kids from 16 different guys will be able to get Pulmicourt repules, Xopenex and Sigular chewable for all 16 kids minor runny noses.

My first thought upon reading this was an uncontrollable urge to raise taxes. That way we could afford to adequately fund our public schools so someday I could stop getting comments with such disregard for the rules of grammar and spelling of the English language. A customer then interrupted me to ask if I could help him put a stamp on a letter. Weird. When I was done I read the hate mail again and then I saw it. I read the message one more time to be sure. Yes. A connection to my very soul was being made.

    I read the message a fourth and fifth time. What was so mesmerizing was how the words were obviously written just for me. The way AJ, the person who cared enough to write, didn't just spit up the same right wing drool that one can hear up and down the AM radio dial, see on Fox news, read in The Wall Street Journal or hear wherever middle aged white people talk amongst themselves. AJ carefully took my thoughts and by adding his own unique, personal take on what I had written, was able to show me the error of my ways in a way Rush Limbaugh or Bill O'Reilly or the guys down at the elks lodge never could. Thank you AJ. Thanks to your intervention I now realize:

1) The fact I own property in the most insane real estate market in the country and drive a two year old paid for car are signs that I am being taxed to death.

2) That social services are the only thing the government spends tax dollars on. It really was a relief to find out that the war in Iraq, a war that I despise, a war that I hate with every past, current and future living part of me, did not cost us a single dollar. Maybe Bush Sr. got a "buy one get one free" special on the first Gulf War. Republicans are smarter that the rest of you, and since I've only been one for about 5 minutes, I'll leave it up to them to explain how the free war thing works.

3) There is no such thing as a rich slut. That the fact Paris Hilton doesn't have 16 different kids by 16 different guys has nothing to do with the fact liberals have fought for a woman's right to contraception access.

I feel like AJ has removed the cataracts from my eyes, but also foolish for having wasted so many years taxing myself to death. I vow to you now dear reader, that I will make up for lost time. That I, the Drugmonkey, will so help me God turn this book into every tax and spend hippie fornicator's worst nightmare.

Let's get started.

My Time As A Republican, Part Two

I'm a little nervous, you know, 180 degree turn in political philosophy and all, but here goes.

I don't understand why poor people hate America so much. I mean Jesus Christ, I wish I was poor. The dream homes of south central Los Angeles, the opportunity to live amongst the high society of Crips and Bloods, the glamour of waiting in line for food stamps. Yet all these ungrateful schmucks can do is gripe about how tired they are after working 2 seven dollar an hour jobs for 12 hours a day, or how they want an apartment without cockroaches. Hell, when I was a kid we couldn't afford ANY pets!

And what's the deal with all these illegal immigrants? Coming across the desert in caravans of air-conditioned Hummers to take all our jobs. Just yesterday they fired the pharmacist I worked with and replaced her with some guy named Javier. Javier doesn't speak English very well, but from what I understand, he told me he made the 2,000 mile trip from Oaxaca because he got bronchitis and he heard he could get a free asthma inhaler in the US. He also said he wasn't willing to take any job that didn't pay at least $80,000 a year, and that 3 other people that snuck across the border with him now work as supermodels. Another is the CEO of Proctor and Gamble. Any intelligent person can see we must stop these immigrants to protect our way of life.

What I really need right now is a tax cut.

And the gay people. Don't even get me started on the gay people. What's with them coming up to me out of the blue and proposing marriage? Every time I try to go to the grocery store there's some mustached Freddy Mercury look alike there wearing a wedding gown asking me to radically alter the institution of matrimony. Obviously this is a part of the wider homosexual agenda Jerry Falwell kept telling me about. If the gays aren't stopped then the terrorists have won, that's what I say, and if you don't think like me, then you're a liberal terrorist that hates America just like poor people do.

Oh, and my tax cut. If I don't get my tax cut the terrorists have won too.

The LSD Wears Off And Ends My Time In The GOP

Oh man, I should have known something was up when the balding, middle aged, paunchy white guy asked me to lick the stamp for his letter. Said his Viagra was giving him a dry mouth and he really needed to get this in the mail. Evidently it was his idea of a sick joke to slip the pharmacist some acid right before closing time. You wouldn't believe the things I saw. My hand melted. Caravans of Mexican supermodels were crossing the desert in Hummers with the air conditioning cranked. The lead Hummer was driven by a guy in a suit with a head that looked like a box of Tide. Freddy Mercury was in front of a Safeway wearing a wedding dress. Weird shit man. Thank God it was just some sort of bad dream.

I'm gonna go sleep this off and be happy my hands are back

Lloyd Duplantis. Worst Scientist Ever.

As the pre-sellout Bono would have said, I could not believe the news that day, but there it was, being broadcast across the country on almost 200 National Public Radio stations and around the world via internet. The topic on host Tom Ashbrook's show *On Point* that night was "Pharmacists and Conscience," a growing trend of pharmacists who refused to dispense birth-control or morning after pills. I found the whole premise of the show a bit surprising as I drove home along the California coast that night. I never thought we would be having this kind of discussion in 21st century America, at least not among my colleagues, educated professionals who should know that the medical definition of when pregnancy begins is the moment a fertilized egg implants into the uterus. People who should know that this definition was adopted because it is not uncommon in nature for a fertilized egg to fail to do this, making defining the beginning of pregnancy as the moment of conception useless to science.

Let me repeat, it is not the moment of fertilization that science recognizes as the beginning of a pregnancy. It is the moment of implantation.

One of the guests on *On Point* that night however, was a pharmacist named Lloyd Duplantis. Lloyd said he refused to sell oral contraceptives "in the name of science" claiming they were "the most dangerous chemical on the market"

More dangerous evidently than the anti-acne medicine Accutane, which requires a woman to test negative for pregnancy and to be on two forms of contraception before a prescription can be issued because of devastating birth defects it will cause in a developing fetus.

More dangerous than thalidomide, which was pulled from the European market after babies started showing up with grossly misshapen limbs after exposure to it in the womb. It is back on the market now, available under tightly controlled conditions, but not, according to Lloyd, as dangerous as a birth control pill.

There are also chemotherapy agents on the market that are direct descendants of the mustard gas used in the trenches of World War I. And safer, evidently, than an oral contraceptive.

I'm not saying hormonal contraceptives are risk free. They are not. I covered the association between Ortho-Evra and cardiovascular risks earlier in the book, and while the high doses of estrogen that product puts in the bloodstream make it an extraordinary case, all hormonal contraceptives carry some risk to the cardiovascular system. If you're past your mid-thirties and especially if you're a smoker, you may want to take a good look at other contraceptive options. They also contain estrogen, and I also covered the link between long term estrogen use and breast cancer earlier. Here's a little irony though. Birth control pills do increase a woman's risk for breast cancer while she is taking them, but they lead to an overall 12% reduction of cancer risk over the course of a lifetime.

Let me repeat that. If you've used hormonal contraceptives at some point in your life, you have a lower cancer risk than if you had not, even though you had a slightly higher risk while you were actually taking them. That's what the science says. If that's the most dangerous chemical on the market, than I am very optimistic what we will find out about the least dangerous one. Bottom line: hormonal contraceptives are products used by millions of people so they can have some control over their sex lives, at the risk of increased cardiovascular side effects. A description I could also use, word per word, for Viagra. I wonder if Lloyd Duplantis feels Viagra is too dangerous for his customers. I've never talked to him, but I have a feeling he doesn't. Lloyd Duplantis is either reading the scientific literature in a way that leads him to the exact opposite conclusion of almost everyone else in the scientific community or he is a religious fundamentalist trying to disguise the fact he wants to impose his morality on the world by wrapping his arguments in a lab coat. I'll let you decide which is more likely.

Surprise turned to shock as I listened to Lloyd that night. Having grown up in the rural Midwest, I was well aware there was no shortage of Christian fundamentalists in this country. But it was easy to forget about them once I made my move to liberal coastal California. Years had gone by without anyone asking me if I was saved or being offended by my favorite semi-swear, "Oh, Christ on a cracker." But, they hadn't gone away. They had been mobilizing and organizing and now they seemed ready to storm the gates of my profession, eager to use the trust pharmacists had earned over the course of more than a century to advance their ideological agenda. Lloyd Duplantis was speaking as a pharmacist and of a man of science that night, and I knew there would be people listening who would trust what he was saying because of this.

I couldn't close my eyes and make it go away. Literally, because it was on the radio, and figuratively, because Lloyd Duplantis that night had been granted a larger megaphone than I thought I could ever have. That's why I wrote this book. Hopefully you've been entertained by some whacky customer tales, learned to be a bit more skeptical of the motives of giant pharmaceutical corporations, maybe let out a chuckle or two as you've read about drugstore life and how it can warp the mind, but I really want you to read the next chapter. The next chapter is my contribution to a world where "pro-life" means protecting the interests of people that are actually alive, not keeping the women of the world burdened with children that are unwanted, and if more people see the next chapter in this book than heard Lloyd Duplantis on the radio that night, I will consider myself a success and be able to retire a happy man.

So do me and the world a favor, and keep reading.

Plan B Went From Medical Secret To Household Name, And If I Have My Way, Another Drug Will As Well.

I had been up late the night before. You know by now I am an unapologetic liberal and Michael Moore's latest film, *Capitalism: A Love Story* had just been released. The release of a new Michael Moore movie is like a liberal holiday, and I was in the middle of a soul-sucking work weekend and needed a little pressure release. I ended up socializing afterwards, running up a sleep debt I knew would make Sunday morning no fun. The hell with it though. The release of a new Michael Moore film does not happen every day and I could handle a sleep debt. Sunday's customers just better not give me any crap.

So naturally there was someone waiting for me to unlock the pharmacy as I drug my seriously sleep-deprived ass towards the happy pill room Sunday morning. I sighed to myself. Then I saw she was crying.

She told me she had been raped the night before, and asked if I sold the Plan B "so I can go home and just make this go away"

I almost crapped myself. Here's the thing. There are people who are trained to deal with these types of situations. I am not one of them. I went to school for five years to learn about drugs. This was taking your local community college quarterback and putting him in a game against the Pittsburgh Steelers.

I pulled her over to the counseling area as I heard the phone start to ring. "Of course I can get you the Plan B, but that will only protect you against pregnancy. There are other things to worry about; I can't do anything for you here to help with STD's. You'd need someone with prescribing authority. It would probably be best to go to the emergency room."

She almost visibly winced at the mention of "emergency room" I decided not to play the "preservation of evidence" card. I don't know why. I'M NOT TRAINED IN THESE THINGS!!!!

Was I supposed to call the police? Am I some sort of required reporter? Fuck fuck fuck.....I DON'T KNOW!!!!! I scrambled around in the pocket as Mean Joe Greene bore down to take my head off.

I got the Plan B. I picked the single-pill version. For those of you not in the profession I'll tell you Plan B originally came in a two pill pack, with instructions to take one tablet now and one in 12 hours. It was always an open secret, however, that you could just take both tablets at once and not lose any efficacy. So when Plan B lost its patent the manufacturer came out with a single pill version and got a new patent on that. I knew it would cost her more, but in her mental state I didn't want her to hear one set of

195

instructions from me and see another set printed on the box. I also didn't want her to take one tablet and then flip out for whatever reason and not take the second dose, so the single pill version is what I sold her. I think I completed a forward pass for a few yards with that one, but I'm not really sure.

"I hope you'll still get some medical attention" I said as three phone lines rang and someone was beating on the gate of the drop off window I had yet to open.

"Well, do you think maybe an urgent care?" She asked softly.

"It would definitely be better than nothing" I said, and told her how to get to the good one. "It's a little further away, but the staff there is really good" Which was my way of saying I hoped to hell she would avoid the house of quackery that was nearby. "Let me get you their phone number"

Later, I realized that while I was in the phone book, I easily could have found the number for the rape crisis center as well. Goddamn it. Thrown back for a 20 yard sack.

I rang out the Plan B, gave her the paper with the directions and phone number for the urgent care, looked her in the eye and told her it would be OK. I don't know if I'm supposed to say something like that. She said thanks and walked out the door. I have no idea if she went to the urgent care or jumped off a bridge. I'll probably never see her again. The day before I would have told you I've been at this long enough I could handle anything a customer would ever throw at me. Now I was rattled. Totally rattled. My hands were shaking as I finally opened the gate to face the crowd of foaming at the mouth barbarians that had gathered and was now ready to subject me to all the regular shit that goes on in a retail pharmacy. The barbarians would be in a mood fouler than usual because I was not opening on time.

Later that afternoon my District Manager called demanding to know if the monthly controlled substance inventory was going to be finished by the end of the day.

I drank a half a bottle of scotch that night before I fell asleep. That's not an exaggeration.

But it could have been worse. Had this happened before 2006 that woman would have left the pharmacy empty handed.

Plan B, commonly known as "the morning after pill," made quite a splash when it was approved for over the counter sale that year, but there was nothing new about it. By that time it had been available as a prescription product for almost 6 years, and even then, there was nothing new or special about it. Plan B was simply a high dose of an oral contraceptive that had been on the market for years. When I graduated from college in the early 90's my first job as a pharmacist was at a drugstore across the street from a Planned Parenthood clinic, and it wasn't uncommon to see a prescription for four Ovral tablets, a type of birth control pill, with instructions of two to be taken immediately and two to be taken 12 hours later. This was the exact same drug and dose as is in today's Plan B. For the most part though, in the early 90's, while some in the medical professions knew about emergency contraception, they seemed, in the words of my favorite band The Pixies, to be so hush hush......they were so.....*quiet* about it.

Eventually word got out, a clever marketer realized selling a two-tablet package would be easier than expecting pharmacists to pop out individual pills from birth control packs, and Plan B was born.

This was done over the deafening howls of those who think sex is not a natural part of the human experience. The type of people who seem to get busted for unacceptable recreational activity in airport bathrooms. Clergy you're weary of leaving alone with your children. People of that sort hated Plan B.

Eventually, it was decided Plan B would do more to help women like the customer who was waiting for me that Sunday morning if they could get it without a prescription.

Again, the cries of those who feel sex is something to be hidden and ashamed of warned us of the end of civilization. A deputy commissioner of the FDA during the Bush administration, Janet Woodcock, actually warned that making Plan B over the counter might lead the nation's youth to form "sex based cults" centered around its use. I swear she said that.

Plan B does have its limitations. It's generally effective only if taken within the first 72 hours after sex, and works around 90% of the time. If you take it though, civilization will not end, you will not have a sudden urge to form a sex based cult, and you will not have induced an abortion.

Let me repeat that last line, because it refutes something those bathroom stall type folks love to repeat. Plan B is not an abortion pill. Remember the medical definition of when pregnancy begins? When a fertilized egg attaches itself to the uterus. Until that happens, you are not pregnant. Plan B works in one of two ways. It either 1) Prevents the release on an unfertilized egg from the ovaries, or 2) Prevents the attachment of a fertilized egg to the uterine lining. It has no effect on an established pregnancy, which means Plan B is not an abortion pill.

If you would like an abortion pill though, with a proper prescription, I can give you one. I'm not talking about RU-486, now sold under the brand name Mifeprex. You can only get Mifeprex directly from a doctor's office. If you are past the three day effectiveness window for Plan B though, and your doctor doesn't carry Mifeprex and doesn't want to, there is another option. An option that is in that hush hush......so *quiet* about it phase where the high dose Ovral method that became Plan B found itself in the early 90's.

This One's For You Lloyd Duplantis.

Cytotec. That's the brand name of the anti-ulcer medicine misoprostol that has been around since 1988. Any doctor anywhere in the country can write a prescription for misoprostol, and while it's not as big a seller as it used to be, the chances are pretty good a pharmacy in your town has it on the shelf. Just like any other prescription. Your insurance will cover it. Just like any other prescription, and if you don't have insurance, it should easily cost you less than $30.

It can also be used to induce an abortion. If that's what you want to do, have your doctor write a prescription as follows:

Cytotec 200mcg
#12 tablets
Take as directed

Then take four of the tablets and dissolve them under your tongue. Three hours later dissolve four more, then wait three hours and do it a third time. Another option is to insert four tablets vaginally and repeat with four more in 24 hours. Talk it over with your doctor to decide which way is best for you.

Also, please read the rest of this before you do anything.

First off, let's be clear. Unlike when you take Plan B, you will be ending a viable pregnancy when you take misoprostol. This is an abortion, and if an abortion is not what you want, then you should not take misoprostol.

Misoprostol is not without side effects or risks. The drug works by expelling the fetus, which means you will experience cramps, possibly stronger than anything you've gone through with your period. You can take some over the counter Aleve (naproxen sodium) to help with these cramps if they are troublesome.

You may also experience chills, fever, nausea, vomiting or diarrhea after taking misoprostol. Fever can be treated with naproxen or Tylenol, but if it lasts more than 24 hours you should check with your doctor. Nausea can be treated with over the counter Dramamine.

Misoprostol doesn't always work. It has a success rate of anywhere from 80 to 90%, and there is a chance if it fails it can cause birth defects. You should start to experience bleeding within the first day after taking misoprostol, if no bleeding occurs, then the abortion has failed. Misoprostol should not be used at all after the 9th week of pregnancy due to the risk of excessive bleeding, and should not be used if you have an IUD.

Seek immediate medical attention if, after using misoprostol, you experience heavy bleeding (soaking more than two maxi pads per hour for more than two hours), feel dizzy or lightheaded, or have a fever for more than 24 hours.

If you end up in the hospital, the symptoms will be identical to a spontaneous miscarriage. The medical staff will not know you tried to induce an abortion.

Now you know how you can get an abortion for the cost of a doctor's visit and your prescription co-pay. Do I think it's the best method? No, I don't. Misoprostol combined with Mifeprex is more effective, but I'm aware it won't always be an option, and unlike too many in the medical professions, I think you should be aware of all the options available to you.

And now you are.

One Last Story. How I Became The Pharmacist Who Saved Christmas And Finally Realized Why I Got Into This Profession.

Rage Against The Machine once sang that my anger was a gift, but I never really believed it until that day. I do remember being angry. I was angry because a certain rent-a-doc pulling a shift at the public health clinic had sent his patient to me with a prescription for Prevacid in hand.

Follow me here. Public health clinic = poor people. Not a hard connection to make, but one that seemed beyond the comprehension of the rent-a-doc. Those of you in the profession probably know where I'm going with this. At the time, Prevacid, an anti-ulcer medication, was an incredibly expensive prescription-only product.

I pulled the woman aside. She didn't want to look me in the eye. I tried to speak to her but got only a soft spoken "no habla ingles"

I was mad. I wasn't gonna let this one go. I paged for the janitor to come to the pharmacy to act as a translator.

"Ma'am, this prescription is very expensive...."

"*señora, esta receta es muy caro*"

"She says she'll pay, her husband's stomach really hurts." The janitor really looked kinda annoyed to be doing this. I didn't care. I wasn't letting this one go.

"Ask her if her husband has tried anything that didn't help" On the other side of the pharmacy a wrinkly white dude with a pinkish hue was giving my tech a hard time over why his prescription for Viagra was taking so long to fill.

After a few minutes of misunderstanding she showed me a bottle of store-brand Maalox that "wasn't working anymore."

Those of you in the profession probably know what I did next. The Prevacid was going to cost around $160 a month. A deductible to meet meant she was gonna pay full freight. I grabbed a box of $20 over the counter Prilosec from the antacid aisle and sent word through the translator for the woman's husband to take it regularly for a couple weeks.

Then I went back to work. Another ho-hum moment in an average, ho-hum workday. The main reason I remembered it was because of how much of a dick the pinkish white man was when I got back to the pharmacy. The pinkish white man came very close to being invited to never come back.

The little pink man burned the incident into my memory, but I got a reminder weeks later when I looked up and saw the woman standing in front of me with the janitor.

"She says you're a good doctor" The janitor said. "She bought her son's Christmas present with the money you saved her."

Holy crap. Every once in a while you win one. Twenty years of how much longer, why does it cost so much, where are the paper plates, pointless prior auths, and early narcotic refills, but every once in awhile me and the Cleveland Browns can win one.

The next day I went back to being the health care equivalent of second string Cleveland Brown's left guard Billy Yates, a well compensated, highly trained professional who had to work like hell for the right to become a doormat. I wouldn't be surprised if Billy has a thing for scotch.

But somehow, it felt, different. Like some sort of burden had been lifted from my shoulders. It took awhile to sink in. At first I thought maybe my employer had finally got around to fixing the air conditioning, but a quick check of the thermometer and a recollection that my employer is unwilling to ever spend any money on anything, ever, quickly put that theory to rest. There was definitely some sort of cosmic shift though, a change in the aura that I couldn't quite grasp at first......

....then it hit me like a Mack truck.

"She bought her son's Christmas present with the money you saved her"

My God. The spell of the little plastic stunt motorcycle. It was broken. At long last I was free. I now understood I was put in this place to stop the warping of a young mind. To break the twisted cycle into which I was drawn by never knowing the thrill of seeing a little plastic man on a little plastic motorcycle fly through the air until a little plastic pelvis snapped the way a certain daredevil's did when he tried to jump the fountains at Caesar's Palace. I was born again that day, but I while I was happy to free one child from the clutches of bad toy karma, I knew there was more. By being the anti-Lloyd Duplantis, and actually using what I know to help people, rather than mislead them to further my religious agenda, I could contribute to a world in which every child who is born is wanted and loved. I could help liberate slightly more than half the world's population from a historical tyranny imposed upon them by biology and outdated paternalistic societal norms. Love and liberation, that was my new calling.

And I'll be damned if I can't answer it by using my pharmacy degree. Yes, I now know exactly why I became a pharmacist.

The paper plates, by the way, are on aisle three.

CPSIA information can be obtained at www.ICGtesting.com
Printed in the USA
237008LV00001B/107/P